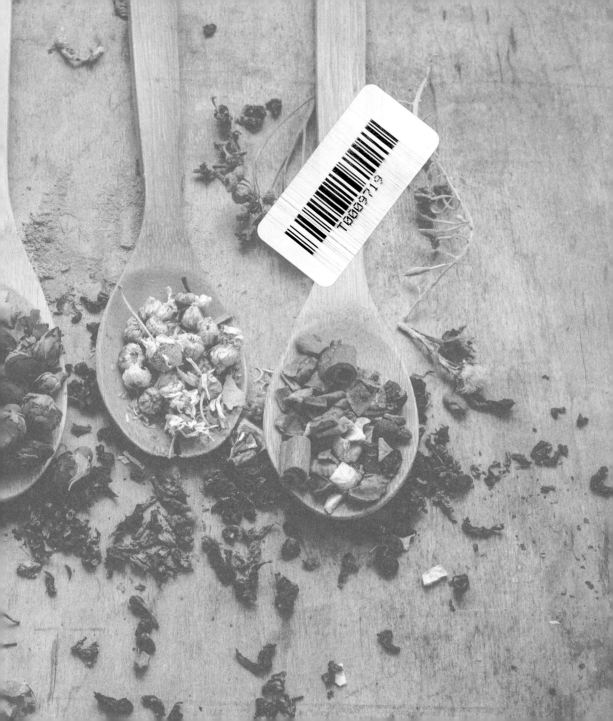

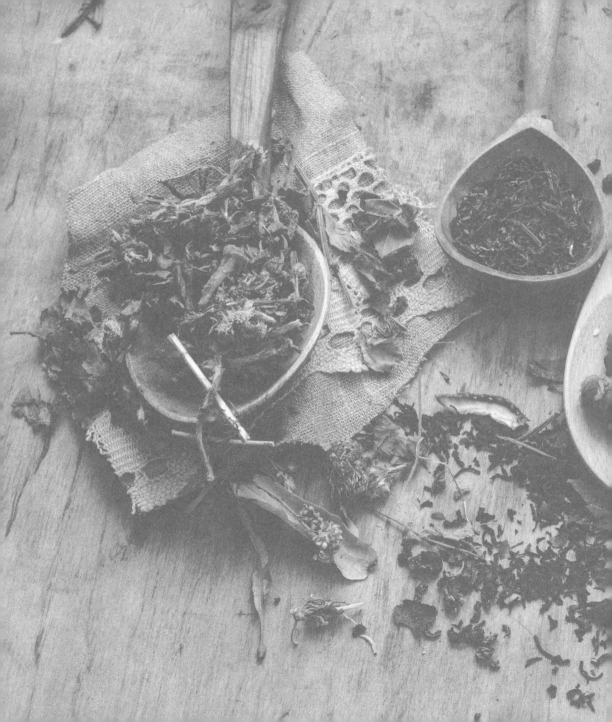

THE
HERBAL
APOTHECARY

THE HERBAL APOTHECARY

An Hachette UK Company
www.hachette.co.uk

Summersdale Publishers Ltd
Part of Octopus Publishing Group Limited
Carmelite House
50 Victoria Embankment
LONDON
EC4Y 0DZ
UK

www.summersdale.com

Printed and bound in China

ISBN: 978-1-80007-985-4

Substantial discounts on bulk quantities of Summersdale books are available to corporations, professional associations and other organizations. For details contact general enquiries: telephone: +44 (0) 1243 771107 or email: enquiries@summersdale.com.

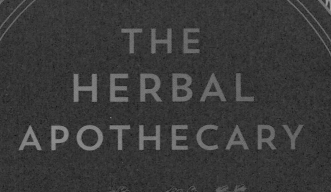

THE
HERBAL
APOTHECARY

RECIPES, REMEDIES
AND RITUALS

CHRISTINE IVERSON

summersdale

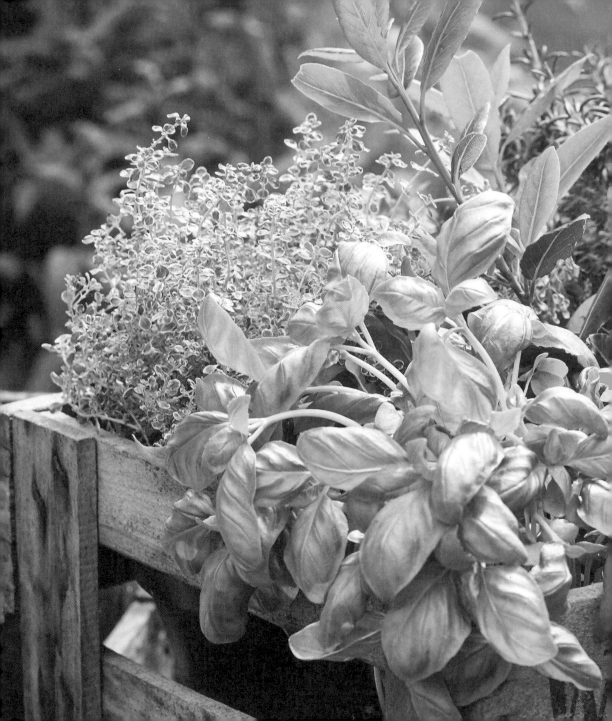

CONTENTS

*Anything is possible if you surround
yourself with the right people.*

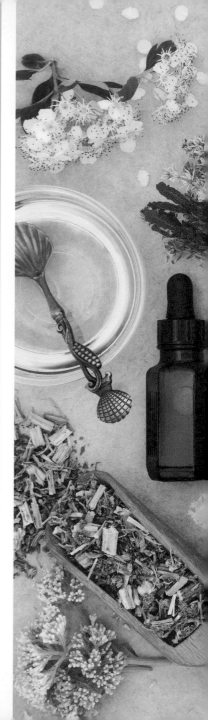

ABOUT THE AUTHOR

Christine Iverson discovered a love of all things herbal after moving to a Sussex downland village in 2001. This fascination led Christine to volunteer as an apothecary at the Weald and Downland Living Museum, where she taught school children about medieval and Tudor medicine. Keen to learn more, she became a regular contributor to her local parish magazine, sharing the folklore and superstitions of herbs with her local community.

Her first book, *The Hedgerow Apothecary*, inspired an undiscovered love of writing and a passion for researching British social history and folk medicine. Taking inspiration from her own back garden, *The Garden Apothecary* and *The Hedgerow Apothecary Forager's Handbook* followed in quick succession, published by Summersdale.

Christine can often be found foraging along the hedgerows and in woodlands with her faithful companion, Rosie the springer spaniel.

INTRODUCTION

"Pay heed to the tales of old wives. It may well be that they alone keep in memory what it was once needful for the wise to know."

J. R. R. Tolkien

My interest in herbs started when I was in infant school, making rose water perfume and potions for my mum from the flowers in our back garden. She was always very appreciative and I realized then how very special it was to be able to create a homemade gift for someone that you love. Since then, herbs have taken over my life, my kitchen cupboards (never throw away an empty bottle or a jar, you never know when you might need it!) and most of the windowsills in my house.

Herbs aren't only plants whose flowers or seeds are valued for their pleasant taste or scent – they also have ample medicinal properties. Creating a simple homemade remedy for a family member with a sore throat or problem skin is such a great skill to learn and one that will set you up for life. Knowing when it's best to seek medical attention is a skill: common sense must be your watchword.

The practice of using plants as medicine dates back thousands of years, with the Ancient Greeks and Romans being the first to record hundreds of types of different herbs and spices and their uses. We have the Roman Empire and its invading forces to thank for introducing the majority of the culinary and medicinal herbs we are familiar with today.

Wise women or cunning folk were to be found in every medieval town or village throughout Europe and were the "go to" people for herbal remedies, potions and charms. This knowledge of plants and their properties was passed down orally from mother to daughter and father to son. Unfortunately, very little was documented in writing because the majority of working people were illiterate at this time.

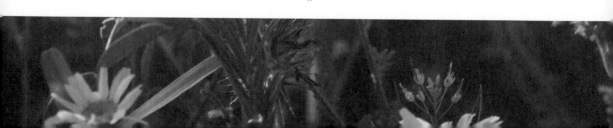

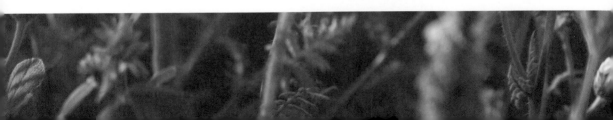

The ascension of King James I to the English throne in 1603 created a culture of suspicion and fear. He was an enthusiastic hunter of "witches" – anyone who administered herbs immediately fell under suspicion and ran the risk of persecution. Sadly, this climate of paranoia led to an immense amount of herb-lore being lost forever, as well as many innocent people being tortured to death.

The one guiding light in this dark period of British history, and a bit of a hero of mine, is the English apothecary Nicholas Culpeper. Unlike his counterparts, who wrote in Latin in order to retain knowledge for themselves, Culpeper wrote his seventeenth-century *Complete Herbal* in English so that anyone, rich or poor, could access medical and pharmaceutical information. To the disapproval of his peers, Culpeper documented hundreds of herbs and spices, along with instructions on how to make simple remedies that ordinary people could follow.

There are many wonderful stories to discover about herbs and their uses throughout history, from prehistoric times through to the Greeks and Romans, right up to the present day – and we are still learning how beneficial they can be. I hope that *The Herbal Apothecary* will summon your ancient "cunning folk" gene and inspire you to incorporate herbs into your everyday life.

This book is intended to be both enlightening and entertaining – it is NOT intended to provide medical advice. It is vital that you take personal responsibility for your own safety when using these remedies. Many herbs and spices should not be used during pregnancy, on babies and small children or by people with certain medical conditions. Always carry out a patch test before putting things on skin or hair in case of allergic reactions. Consult your GP if you have any doubts and always do your research thoroughly.

PREPARING BOTANICALS

It's important to prepare fresh botanicals before infusing them into carrier oils; excess moisture in the plants can turn the oil rancid, rendering it useless. You don't need equipment like dehydrators to prepare your herbs and flowers. I use a piece of chicken wire fashioned into a frame for drying flower heads and petals. Herbs and flowers don't have to be absolutely dry, but they do need to be "wilted" for a couple of hours to remove some of the moisture. Lay petals and leaves onto kitchen paper overnight – whole flower heads will take a bit longer. Bunches of woody herbs can be hung up in cool airy places like outhouses or garden sheds; avoid the kitchen, as they can absorb the cooking smells and smoke.

HERBS

Herbs are at their best before they begin to flower. Harvest them mid-morning on a dry day before the sun has burned away the flowers' essential oils.

- Remove any old, dead or diseased leaves. There's no need to wash them if you grow without the use of pesticides. Give them a gentle shake to remove any insects.

- Tie the herbs into loose bundles with natural twine, hang upside down and put a brown paper bag over them to catch leaves as they dry.

- Keep them away from direct sunlight and leave for at least two weeks or until the leaves are crunchy. It's important that your herbs are completely dry or they could be spoiled by mould growth – check on them regularly and discard any that smell musty or have fluffy mould growing on them.

- Crumble the herbs with your fingers and store in an airtight container, where they will keep for about a year. I've found that rubbing the dried herbs through a colander effectively removes any woody stalks and crumbles the leaves up finely as well.

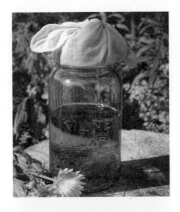

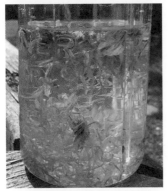

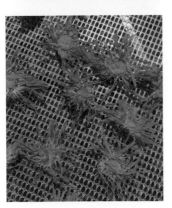

FLOWERS AND PETALS

Harvest flower heads and petals mid-morning on a dry day when the flowers are looking their best. Avoid drying in direct sunlight as this can destroy the very health-giving properties that you wish to harness in your remedies. All you need for the drying process is a flat surface that allows air to circulate freely; chicken wire is perfect for this. Alternatively, hang up some muslin to create a flat hammock, or even use an old wire shelf from the oven. I place my chicken wire tray under the shade of a big old apple tree in the garden on a dry day, although if it's windy you might lose a few flowers. Remember to bring them back inside before nightfall, otherwise the flowers will get damp with the morning dew.

- Lay baking paper over the wire of your drying surface, to prevent smaller petals falling through the gaps.

- Spread petals across the surface in a single layer, trying not to overlap them. They will dry quite quickly.

- Place flower heads far enough apart so they don't touch – these will take a while longer. They will shrivel and become crumbly as they dry. Place in a cool, airy place away from direct sunlight and turn them over occasionally.

- When they feel crunchy and crumble easily, store in an airtight container, label and date. Depending on the drying environment and type of flower, they can take anything from two to four weeks to dry completely. Flower heads and petals will keep for up to a year.

CHOOSING THE RIGHT CARRIER OIL

There are a wide variety of plant-based carrier oils available on the market, all with different beneficial properties. These are used in homemade infused oils, lotions, massage oils and balms; they also "carry" essential oils that need to be diluted before going onto the skin. You can use many of the oils that you have in your kitchen larder or there are a huge variety of sellers online. Try and find one that is reputable and stocks good quality oils – remember this product will be absorbed into your skin and into your bloodstream.

Many oils are pressed from nuts, seeds and kernels. If you have any allergies, make sure you research thoroughly before using them, and always do a patch test first.

TYPE OF OIL	PROPERTIES	HAIR/SCALP		SKIN	
		Oily	Dry	Oily	Dry
Almond	Moisturizing Antioxidant High in vitamin E Natural SPF Nourishing	✓	✓	✓	✓
Apricot kernel	Easily absorbed Antioxidant Anti-ageing Antiseptic High in vitamin A	X	✓	X	✓
Avocado	Soothing Hydrating Natural SPF Antioxidant Anti-inflammatory	X	✓	✓	✓

TYPE OF OIL	PROPERTIES	HAIR/SCALP		SKIN	
		Oily	Dry	Oily	Dry
Coconut	Easily available Antioxidant Anti-inflammatory Anti-microbial Anti-ageing Promotes hair growth	X	✓	X	✓
Grapeseed	High in vitamin E Easily absorbed Antibacterial Antioxidant Anti-dandruff	✓	✓	✓	✓
Jojoba	Antiseptic Hypoallergenic Hydrating Anti-inflammatory Antifungal Anti-acne Healing	✓	✓	✓	✓
Olive	Easily available Skin brightening Antioxidant Anti-ageing Collagen boosting Cleansing	X	✓	✓	✓
Peach kernel	Easily absorbed High in vitamin E Hypoallergenic Good for older skin	X	✓	X	✓
Sunflower	Easily available Anti-inflammatory Moisturizing Easily absorbed	✓	✓	✓	✓

HOW TO MAKE INFUSED CARRIER OILS

Creating infused carrier oils is a lovely way to harness the properties of your garden flowers and herbs and turn them into the wonderful lotions, balms and salves contained in this book. I particularly love to make calendula-infused carrier oil – not only does it become the most beautiful golden orange colour, it also has wonderful skin-healing benefits.

SUN METHOD

Healers and apothecaries have used this traditional method for hundreds of years. Although it takes time and relies heavily on the appearance of the sun, this is definitely my preferred way. I just love to see jars of different coloured botanical oils working their magic and infusing on my south-facing windowsill.

INGREDIENTS

Herbs or flowers
(these can be
dried or fresh)

Carrier oil of
your choice

Equipment needed

Sterilized glass jar

Muslin square

String or elastic band

METHOD

Fill the jar halfway with your plant material.

Cover with your chosen carrier oil, shaking to burst any bubbles. Ensure that all plant material is completely covered – anything sticking out could go mouldy.

Top with the muslin and secure with string or an elastic band.

Place on a sunny windowsill for at least two weeks until the oil has taken on some colour and scent.

Strain the oil through the muslin, squeezing to extract all the oil. Compost the plant material left behind.

Label and date – you might think that you'll remember which oil it is, but believe me you won't!

Keep in a cool dark place and use within a year.

QUICK INFUSION METHOD

In the winter months this technique enables you to infuse carrier oil without the help of the sun. This method is a lot quicker than the sun method, but may not extract as many beneficial oils as the traditional method. Be careful not to fry your plant material by heating the oil too much.

INGREDIENTS

Herbs or flowers (these can be dried or freshly wilted)

Carrier oil of your choice

Equipment needed

Heatproof bowl

Saucepan

Boiling water

METHOD

Put the plant material and carrier oil into your heatproof bowl suspended over the pan of boiling water; ensure the water doesn't touch the bottom of the bowl.

Simmer gently, without a lid, for 2 hours, checking the water level in the pan regularly.

Allow to cool, strain, label and date.

Keep in a cool dark place and use within a year.

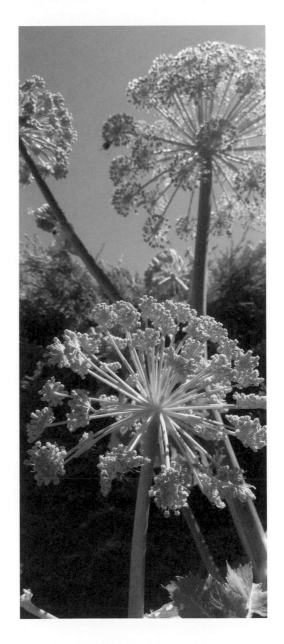

KITCHEN ESSENTIALS

You don't have to spend a fortune on specialist kitchenware; you can manage well with basic cooking utensils and a little ingenuity. A few large pans are essential, a sieve and colander, and some cotton muslin – although a clean cotton tea towel will work well, too. A pestle and mortar if you have one, or a food processor, will make life easier. Jam jars and bottles of differing sizes can be new or recycled, as long as the lids are clean and undamaged, and handwritten labels always look lovely.

Carrier oils: These can be almond oil (don't use if you have a nut allergy), peach kernel oil or even olive oil. These are easily available online and in some health food shops.

HOW TO STERILIZE JARS AND BOTTLES

1. Wash the jars and lids thoroughly in hot soapy water and rinse.

2. Lay the jars in a preheated oven 140°C (280°F) for 10–15 minutes until dry.

3. Soak the lids in boiling water in a bowl, then dry thoroughly with kitchen paper before use.

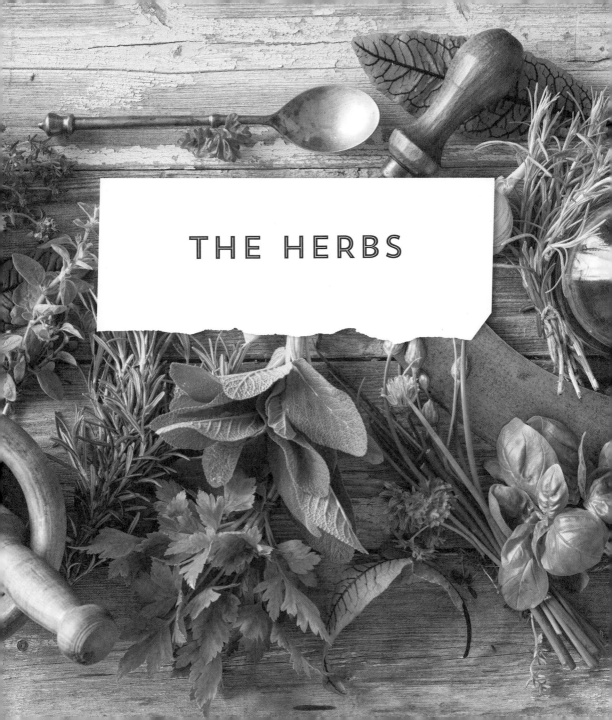

THE HERBS

STARTING A HERB GARDEN

Herbs really are the most wonderful plants to grow in your garden, not just for their medicinal and culinary properties, but because pollinators love them. Many herbs also grow well in pots or on windowsills, so you don't even need a garden to enjoy their benefits.

CHOOSING YOUR HERBS

Think about which herbs you'd like to grow and consider where they will need to be planted – herbs, like many plants, will not thrive in the wrong environment. Some, like the mint family, are incredibly invasive and will choke out other plants if you leave them unchecked. Most herbs are Mediterranean in origin and therefore like to grow in a sunny sheltered spot. I like to grow them by my south-facing patio so that I can enjoy their aroma while having a morning cup of tea – and they are handy to harvest because they are close to my kitchen.

ANNUAL HERBS

These herbs only last for one growing season, but you can easily harvest their seeds to grow them again, year after year. Annual herbs include basil, coriander and parsley.

PERENNIAL HERBS

With a little care these herbs will keep growing all through the year. Perennial herbs include rosemary, thyme and members of the mint family.

MY TOP TEN FAVOURITE HERBS

- **Basil:** This herb likes good drainage and full sun. It is very sensitive to cold and will die in the slightest frost. The great thing about basil is that the more you pick it, the more it grows – and it smells absolutely incredible.

- **Calendula:** Calendula is easy to grow, self-seeding and brings sunshine into the garden. The yellow and orange blooms will last well into the autumn and can be picked and dried for use in your own herbal apothecary.

- **Chives:** This is one of the easiest herbs to grow and can be harvested as soon as 60 days after sowing the seed. Chives have the prettiest of purple flowers, which can add a pop of colour to even the simplest of green salads.

- **Coriander:** Water your coriander sparingly or it could grow too fast and go to seed prematurely. Young coriander plants are a particular favourite of slugs and snails, so make sure that you protect them with cloches or netting.

- **Lavender:** I grow lavender on my patio, mainly for its wonderful scent, but also because the bees just love it. Lavender doesn't like being in cold, damp, shady spots, preferring free-draining soil and full sun.

- **Mint:** This herb comes in many varieties including apple mint, basil mint and even chocolate mint. Beware: mint is a bit of a bully and will spread rapidly if planted in the ground – pop it into a pot to contain its vigour.

- **Oregano:** This herb likes hot, dry conditions and free-draining soil. Oregano flowers are very attractive to pollinators, while the leaves are delicious in a variety of Italian dishes.

- **Rosemary:** A delightful evergreen shrub which can last long into the autumn and beyond if given well-drained sandy soil and lots of sunlight. Rosemary likes to be pruned – cutting it regularly for kitchen use will be sufficient.

- **Sage:** Not all varieties of sage are edible – choose garden sage or golden sage if you want to cook with this herb. Sage doesn't like to have its roots sitting in water, so make sure to choose well-drained soil or to plant it in a container with lots of grit.

- **Thyme:** Lemon thyme is my personal favourite; I just love the citrusy scent and flavour. Other varieties include common thyme, woolly thyme and lavender thyme, as well as many others. They all enjoy well-drained soil and lots of sun. Pollinators will also be drawn to the tiny aromatic flowers.

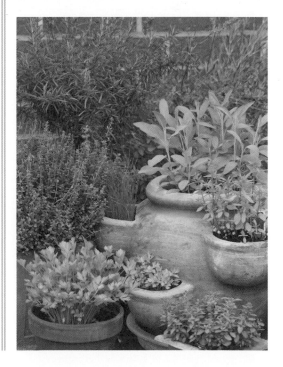

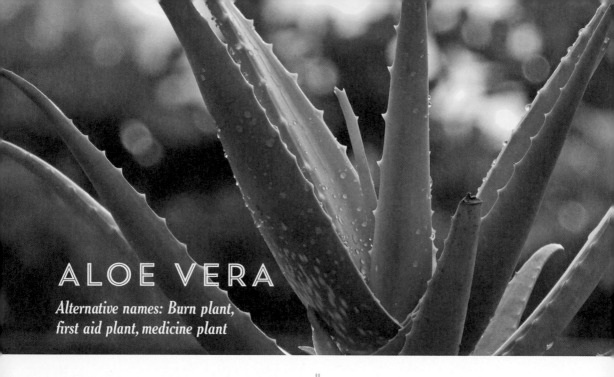

ALOE VERA

*Alternative names: Burn plant,
first aid plant, medicine plant*

HOW TO IDENTIFY: Although this herb is native to the hot climes of Africa, Madagascar and the Arabian Peninsula, in cooler climates aloe vera can be successfully grown on warm windowsills and in greenhouses if it is protected from frost. A member of the succulent family, aloe vera has thick, fleshy, pointed leaves with little "teeth" along the edges.

HISTORY: Thousands of years ago, Egyptian queens Cleopatra and Nefertiti are both known to have used the nourishing juice of aloe vera in their beauty routines. Aloe vera was also used in the embalming process for its antibacterial and antifungal properties.

The Knights Templar drank aloe juice with palm wine and hemp – a concoction they called the "Elixir of Jerusalem" – believing that it would add years to their lives.

The fifteenth-century explorer Christopher Columbus grew aloe vera plants on board his ships to use medicinally as a wound healer. At the same time, indigenous Americans referred to the aloe vera plant as "the wand of heaven", applying it to their skin for its healing and moisturizing properties, as well as to wooden cooking and working implements in order to prevent insect infestation.

During the Second World War, aloe juice provided by botanical gardens was used to heal radiation burns caused by X-rays.

Pilgrims to Mecca still hang aloe over the doorways of their homes as a protective measure, as well as to symbolize that they are performing Hajj.

FOLKLORE: In South American culture, aloe leaves are strung round the house to ward off evil spirits, keep members of the household safe from accidents and to ensure good luck.

FOLK MEDICINE: Pliny the Elder, a commander in the Roman army, naturalist and author of *Naturalis Historia*, recommended that aloe juice be used to cure the sores of leprosy and to reduce perspiration. It is also known as the "first aid plant" and "medicine plant"; these names are indicative of the respect that was given to aloe vera and its healing properties.

In the seventeenth century, Culpeper described how:

"Aloes made into powder, and strewed upon bloody wounds, stops the blood and heals them [...] boiled with wine and honey it heals rifts and haemorrhoids [...] removes obstructions of the viscera, kills worms in the stomach and intestines."

OTHER COMMON USES: An aloe leaf can be cut open to reveal the gel inside. This can then be rubbed onto minor burns to give instant relief and speed up the healing process.

Aloe is very skin friendly and is therefore used widely in cosmetics and sun creams. I'm sure many of you had bitter aloes painted on your fingernails as a child to deter biting – I certainly did.

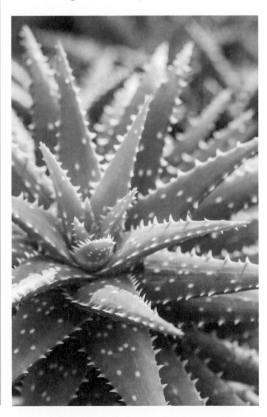

ALOE VERA FACIAL TONER

Making natural products to use on your body can be hugely beneficial, not only because they leave your skin soft and glowing, but because it can also be good for your bank balance. Free from chemicals, parabens and other nasties, this aloe vera toner is suitable for all skin types. It restores the natural pH of your skin and is so easy to make that you'll soon be gifting it to friends and family, too.

Makes approx. 100 ml

INGREDIENTS

90 ml organic rose water

1 tbsp organic aloe vera gel

2 tbsp distilled witch hazel (available at the chemist)

5 drops rose essential oil

5 drops camomile essential oil

Equipment needed

Blender

Sieve

Sterilized bottle

TO MAKE THE ROSE WATER

Gather three handfuls of pesticide-free rose petals from your garden or another organic source. Pop them into a pan with just enough filtered water to cover.

Bring to the boil, cover and simmer gently for 30 minutes. The petals will lose their colour and it should smell divine.

Strain the liquid into a clean bottle and compost the petals if you can.

Alternatively, rose water can be purchased online or found in the baking aisle of some supermarkets.

TO MAKE THE ALOE VERA GEL

Cut one large aloe leaf from the plant and wash thoroughly.

Cut down the prickly edges of the leaf and then use a sharp knife or your fingers to separate the interior clear gel from the green outsides. The interior gel is what you need.

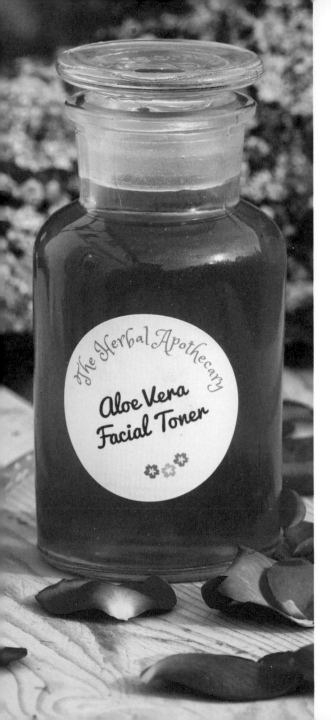

Put the gel into a sieve and allow the yellow sap to drain away, leaving a clear gel.

Cut the clear gel into chunks and then pop these into a blender to create a smooth liquid gel. Strain to remove the pulp.

Alternatively, aloe vera gel can be purchased from health food outlets and larger pharmacies.

METHOD

Mix together the rose water, aloe gel and witch hazel in a small jug.

Add the essential oils and mix.

Pour the mixture into a clean bottle.

Shake well before use and sweep gently over the skin with a cotton pad.

Kept refrigerated, this facial toner should last a month.

Always do a patch test first.

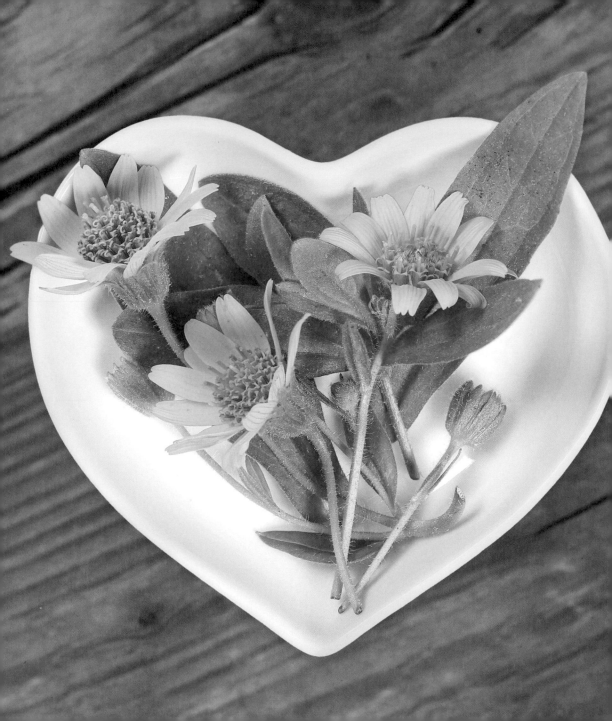

ARNICA

Alternative names: Wolf's bane, leopard's bane, mountain tobacco

HOW TO IDENTIFY: The word arnica comes from the Greek *"arni"*, meaning lamb. This is probably a reference to the plant's fluffy leaves, stems and flowers. This perennial herb has yellow daisy-like flowers that come into bloom in late spring and early summer.

Arnica can be found growing in the sandy soil of the mountains of North America, as well as in the Alps and Pyrenees in northern Europe.

HISTORY: The first known use of arnica can be traced back to the early sixteenth century, when it was a popular German folk remedy used to treat blunt injuries, bruising, inflammation and skin lesions.

German goat herders noticed that their animals would clamber up the mountains in search of arnica flowers to eat in order to heal themselves after falling or stumbling. Arnica is called *"fallkraut"* in German, meaning "fall herb".

FOLKLORE: One European superstition claimed that planting arnica around a cornfield would keep the spirit of the Corn Wolf penned there. He would then wander around the fields, adding his strength to the coming harvest. Finally, his spirit would enter the last sheaf of corn, which would then be cut and carried proudly aloft by the villagers.

To prevent violent thunderstorms, arnica can be burned while saying, "Arnica bright, arnica alight. Thunderstorm, turn and take flight."

To protect your home and bring fertility to your garden, arnica should be sprinkled around the boundaries of your property.

FOLK MEDICINE: The first medical reference to arnica is believed to have come from the writings of the twelfth-century German abbess Hildegard of Bingen. Here she recommends that: *"If spots and blisters erupt between the skin and flesh, then let the person cook the herb in water and wrap the blemishes, and then the person will be healed."*

A hair rinse made with arnica extract was believed to treat hair loss caused by anxiety or stress.

OTHER COMMON USES: To relieve tired, sore feet, add a few drops of arnica tincture to warm water for a footbath.

ARNICA AND MATCHA LOTION BAR

Lotion bars are such a joy to make because you can use all sorts of pretty moulds to turn them into special gifts. Arnica is well known for its anti-inflammatory properties; matcha tea is antibacterial; peppermint oil is cooling and analgesic; and shea butter will leave your skin silky smooth.

Makes approx. two 60-ml lotion bars

INGREDIENTS

35 ml arnica-infused carrier oil (see page 14)

35 g organic shea butter

45 g unrefined beeswax

20 drops peppermint essential oil

1 tsp matcha green tea powder

Equipment needed

Silicone moulds or cupcake cases

METHOD

Melt the arnica-infused carrier oil, shea butter and beeswax in a heatproof bowl placed over a pan of boiling water.

Once melted, take the mixture off the heat and stir in the essential oil and matcha. Try not to create any bubbles, because these can spoil the look of your finished lotion bar.

Pour into silicone moulds if you have them. Alternatively, you can use cupcake cases or any other small flexible containers that you have around the kitchen.

Allow the mixture to cool completely before popping the lotion out of the mould.

These lotion bars will melt as they are rubbed gently onto the skin.

Only use this product on unbroken skin and always do a patch test first. Do not use if allergic to the daisy family. Not recommended during pregnancy or while breastfeeding.

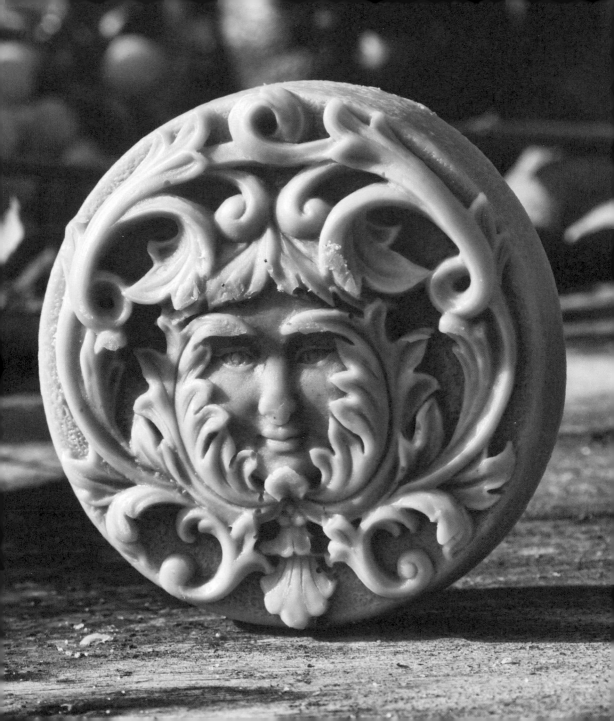

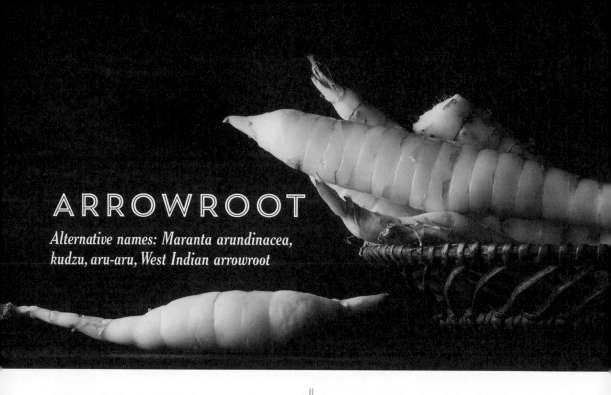

ARROWROOT

Alternative names: Maranta arundinacea, kudzu, aru-aru, West Indian arrowroot

HOW TO IDENTIFY: Arrowroot is a starch traditionally obtained from the rhizomes of the tropical *Maranta arundinacea* plant. This herb can be found in powdered form on most supermarket shelves.

HISTORY: The Arawak people of South America first cultivated arrowroot for use as a food starch and medicine as early as 5000 BCE. It was so valued for its healing properties that it was nicknamed *aru-aru*, meaning meal of meals.

Indigenous Americans are believed to have introduced arrowroot plants to the Caribbean. European colonists then became the main exporters of the herb in the eighteenth century, the majority of it making its way to Britain in the form of flour.

Arrowroot flour was one of the four main medicinal remedies carried by nineteenth-century Antarctic explorers, who used it for its anti-inflammatory properties and also to help relieve diarrhoea.

FOLKLORE: According to folklore, this tropical perennial was used by the inhabitants of Central America to heal the wounds of warriors injured by poison arrows.

Dust your hands with arrowroot powder to bring good luck in games of chance, or use it to treat gangrene, spider bites and scorpion stings.

FOLK MEDICINE: The first known use of arrowroot by European colonists was as a treatment for sores and infections, where slices of the tuber were placed directly on the skin.

This herb was also widely used in cakes, puddings and sauces. Arrowroot was historically used to treat babies with diarrhoea, and biscuits made with the flour soothed sore gums during teething.

By the 1920s, arrowroot was being marketed as "invalid food", because it is a safe ingredient unlikely to upset the stomachs of even the youngest children. One British recipe from *Cooking for Invalids – Recipes for the Bedridden* by Phyllis Browne, published in the nineteenth century, recommends that "*Half a pint of milk, one ounce of arrowroot, one ounce of caster sugar*" be prepared as follows: "*Mix the arrowroot smoothly with a little cold milk; boil the rest of the milk and stir in the arrowroot; stir and boil well, taking care it does not burn*". Sounds very similar to custard to me.

OTHER COMMON USES: The binding properties of arrowroot make it a great substitute for eggs. Just 2 tbsp of arrowroot mixed with 3 tbsp of water can replace one large egg in baking or in omelettes.

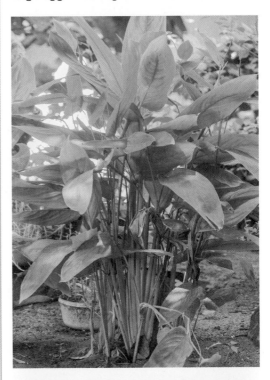

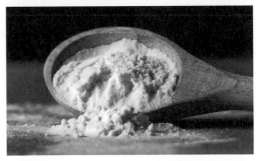

ARROWROOT AND COCONUT TOOTHPASTE

The anti-inflammatory properties of arrowroot can help to soothe sore gums, making it the perfect ingredient in toothpaste. Bicarbonate of soda is a natural whitener; coconut oil binds with any bacteria, which will then be discarded at the end of teeth cleaning; and sea salt can help neutralize acid in the mouth.

Makes approx. 80 ml

INGREDIENTS

½ tsp fine sea salt

2 tsp bicarbonate of soda

4 tbsp room temperature organic coconut oil

1–2 tsp organic arrowroot powder

3 drops peppermint essential oil

Equipment needed

Sterilized tin or jar

METHOD

Add the salt and bicarbonate of soda to the coconut oil and mix thoroughly.

Start by stirring in 1 tsp of arrowroot powder. Add the rest of the arrowroot powder if your toothpaste doesn't seem thick enough.

Incorporate the peppermint oil until it has been evenly distributed throughout the paste.

Pop your toothpaste into a sterilized tin or jar.

This toothpaste will keep for about three weeks. To minimize contamination of your toothpaste, use a small spoon to add the paste to your toothbrush.

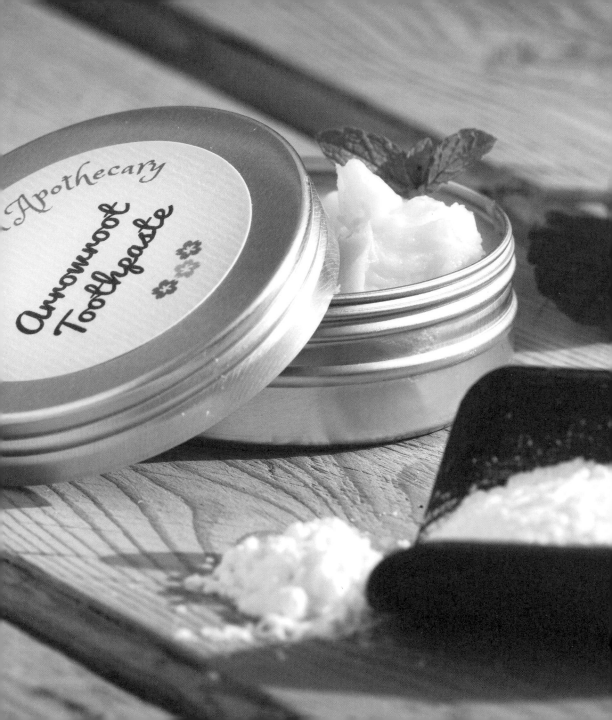

BASIL

Alternative names:
St Joseph's wort, holy basil,
sweet basil, king of herbs

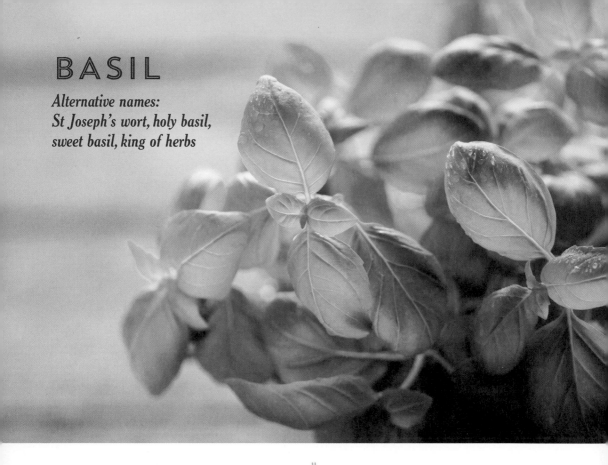

HOW TO IDENTIFY: Common basil is a tender herb with glossy green leaves and a peppery-liquorice flavour and scent.

HISTORY: The herb originated in South East Asia, and we can thank the Romans for introducing basil to European kitchens and medicine cabinets. Pliny recommends this herb as an aphrodisiac, not just for people, but for horses and donkeys, too.

The Ancient Greeks strangely believed that to grow particularly fragrant basil you should shout and swear angrily as you sow the seeds into the ground.

In India it was believed that a basil leaf placed on the tongue would aid the passage of the dead to heaven. It was also considered so sacred that criminals once had to swear an oath on basil in a court of law.

FOLKLORE: In Roman mythology, the Basilisk was a fire-breathing dragon that could kill you just by looking at you. Luckily, basil was just the antidote you needed to counteract the Basilisk's venom.

The Ancient Greeks used basil to detect witches. They called out the names of suspected witches while burning basil and if the leaves crackled on one particular name, the person in question was undoubtedly a witch.

It was believed that smelling basil would cause scorpions to grow in your brain, and placing basil under a stone and waiting for two days would turn it into a scorpion! In the fourth century, Hilary of Poitiers, a French Doctor of the Church, asserted that an acquaintance of his experienced a *"scorpion bred in his brain"* after smelling basil. Even Culpeper believed that *"being laid to rot in horse dung, [basil] will breed venomous beasts"*.

Basil will shrivel in the hands of an unfaithful wife. However, carrying it on your person will bring you good luck and wealth.

In seventeenth-century England, basil was hung above doorways and strewn on the floor to ward off evil spirits, according to the adage *"where basil lays no evil can enter"*.

FOLK MEDICINE: Basil is analgesic and a muscle relaxant. As such, it is especially effective on tension headaches and sinus pain when inhaled from a steam bath.

OTHER COMMON USES: Basil is the perfect companion plant for tomatoes, not just because the two cook beautifully together, but also because it keeps away tomato hornworms, aphids and whitefly.

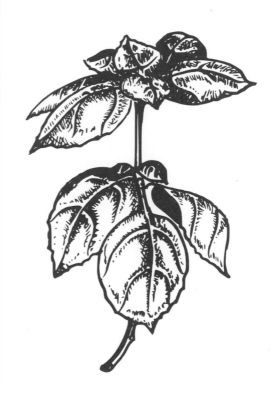

FRAGRANT BASIL SALT

Once you have made plenty of pesto for freezing, this is a great way to preserve basil from your garden. Use basil sea salt to season foods that pair well with basil such as tomatoes, as a rejuvenating skin scrub or even add it to bath salts to help heal bacterial and fungal infections. Other herbs work equally well in this recipe, so feel free to use whatever you have growing in your garden or on your windowsill.

INGREDIENTS

A good handful of basil leaves

125 g natural sea salt

Equipment needed

Stick blender or food processor

Baking tray

Pestle and mortar or rolling pin

METHOD

Wash the basil leaves and pat dry on a clean tea towel.

Use a stick blender or food processor to blitz the salt and basil together until the herbs are finely chopped.

Spread the basil salt in a thin layer onto a baking tray lined with greaseproof paper and leave to dry naturally away from direct sunlight for 24 hours.

Use a pestle and mortar or the end of a rolling pin to break up any clumps of salt.

Sprinkle a small amount onto sliced heirloom tomatoes, tomato soup, pizza and pasta.

Store in an airtight container for up to four months.

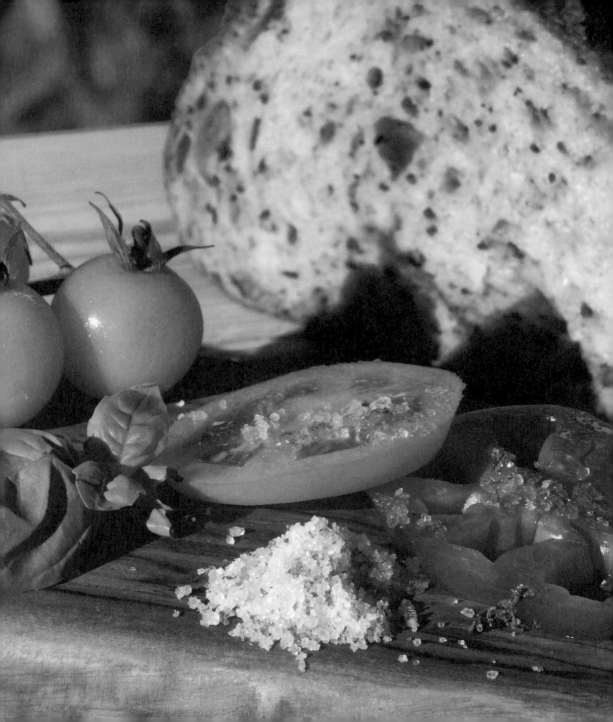

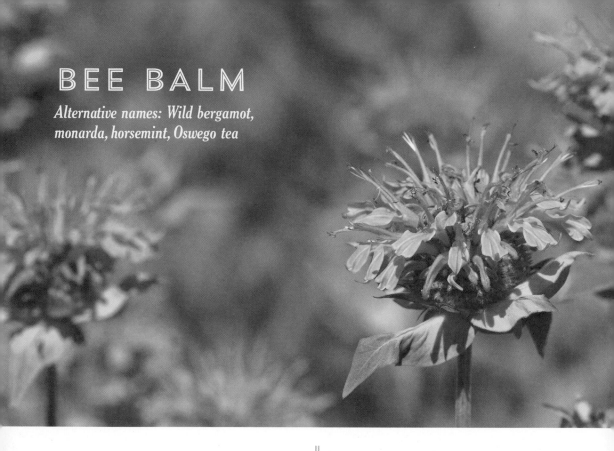

BEE BALM

Alternative names: Wild bergamot, monarda, horsemint, Oswego tea

HOW TO IDENTIFY: As with all members of the mint family, bee balm has a four-sided, slightly hairy square stem. It has scarlet red tubular raggedy flowers that grow to over 3 cm (1 in.) long, as well as leaves that smell like a delicious mix of bergamot orange, thyme and mint.

HISTORY: Eighteenth-century American botanist John Bartram collected some bee balm seeds from Oswego, near New York, and sent them to England. The British loved them, and Oswego tea was soon to be found in Covent Garden, one of London's most famous fruit and vegetable markets.

In 1773, The Sons of Liberty, a clandestine group dedicated to undermining British rule in Colonial America, threw 342 chests of black tea imported by the British into Boston harbour in protest at the high taxes imposed by the British parliament. This event was known as the Boston Tea

Party and ultimately led to the American Revolution in 1775. After the Boston Tea Party, Americans began drinking Oswego tea as a home-grown replacement for imported tea – they didn't want to stop drinking tea, but they certainly didn't want to pay high British taxes either.

FOLKLORE: A tattoo of a bee balm flower will bring the bearer prosperity and good luck.

In floriography, the language of flowers, bee balm symbolizes good health and protection against evil and illness.

Bee balm tied in a cloth and placed under hot running bathwater will bring you peace, contentment and happiness, and will dissipate any negative energies. A spotted variety of bee balm is even believed to ward off ghosts!

FOLK MEDICINE: Bee balm has a high thymol content, which gives it antibacterial properties. It also has antifungal and anaesthetic qualities, making it useful for mouthwashes, foot baths and as a wash for minor cuts and scrapes.

Bergamot tea made from the leaves and flowers is beneficial for fever and stomach problems and can be used as a gentle sleep aid.

Indigenous Americans drank bee balm tea to treat colds and flu and also to bathe wounds and swellings caused by bee stings – hence the name bee balm.

OTHER COMMON USES: Butterflies love bee balm and will be attracted to your garden if you grow it.

The entire above-ground plant is edible, and while some people still brew tea from the leaves, others like to put the colourful flowers into a salad.

Dried leaves smell a little like bergamot orange and are a delightfully scented addition to pot-pourri and drawer sachets.

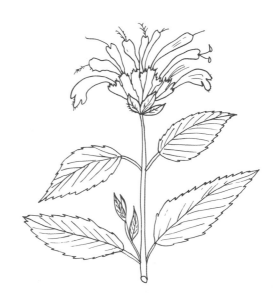

ICED BEE BALM TEA

Bee balm has a soothing effect on the digestive tract and is therefore helpful in the treatment of indigestion and nausea as well as colds and flu. Due to its antispasmodic properties, it can ease menstrual cramps as well as bloating and coughs – it can help to calm the nerves, too.

INGREDIENTS

A small bunch of
pesticide-free bee balm

Filtered water

Honey or fruit syrup
to sweeten

Equipment needed

Sterilized jar

Muslin or tea towel

METHOD

Remove the leaves from the bee balm stems and pick the red petals from the flower heads. Compost the stems if you can.

Fill a clean jar with filtered water.

Add the bee balm leaves and petals and stir well.

Secure the lid and shake.

Place the jar in the fridge for 24 hours, shaking every couple of hours.

Strain the mixture through a muslin or clean tea towel.

Sweeten to taste with honey or fruit syrup.

Serve over ice with a wedge of lemon.

FOR HOT BEE BALM TEA: Infuse the leaves and petals in just-boiled water and allow to steep for 10 minutes.

Not to be taken during pregnancy.

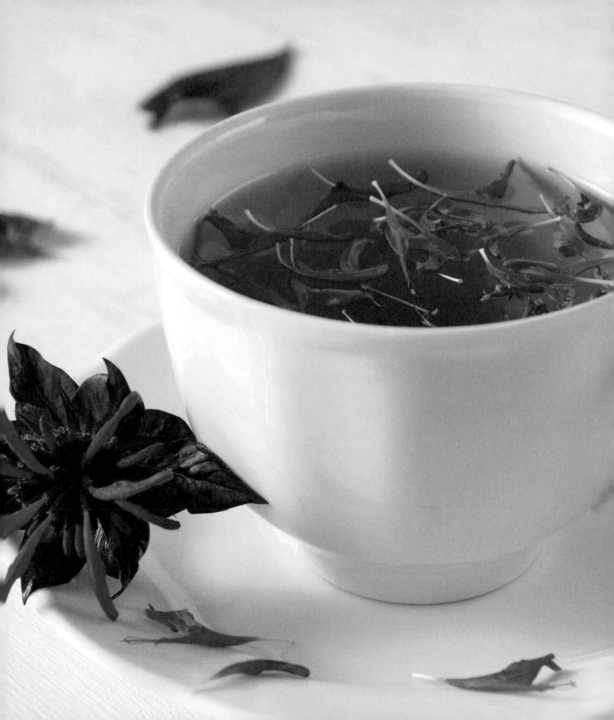

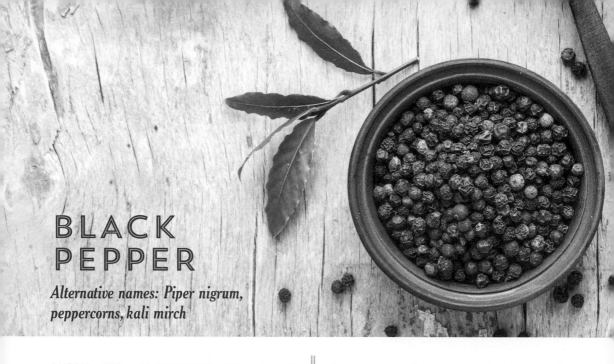

BLACK PEPPER

Alternative names: Piper nigrum, peppercorns, kali mirch

HOW TO IDENTIFY: This plant is cultivated along the west coast of India. Its peppercorns grow on a tall vine that carries clusters of small fruits. These fruits turn from green to orange and then to red as they ripen. For black pepper, green fruits are picked and dried until the whole fruit becomes black and hard. For white pepper, the fruits are dried and just the seeds are used.

HISTORY: Arguably the most commonly used spice in kitchens all over the world, black pepper has a history that dates back thousands of years.

Peppercorns were found in the nostrils of the Egyptian pharaoh Rameses II, put there as part of the mummification ritual in 1213 BCE. Cleopatra was said to have lotions made for her skin using black pepper, while Egyptian toothpaste was made from rock salt, black pepper, mint and iris flowers.

The Ancient Greeks used black pepper mainly for medicinal purposes. Occasionally it was used in wine, but very rarely in food. The Romans, however, discovered a love of cooking with pepper. In fact, three out of four recipes in *De Re Culinaria*, a collection of Roman recipes compiled by Marcus Gavius Apicius in the first century CE, called for this ingredient.

So prized was black pepper that Roman Emperor Domitian built warehouses called "horrea piperataria", specifically for storing pepper and other spices as a precaution against thieves.

Pepper and spices were ground in special mills to be sold in papyrus bags in Vicus Unguentarius, a market street in Rome where sellers of perfume, raw materials and medicines were also traded.

Sixteenth-century sailors were subjected to a "no pockets, no cuffs" dress rule on board ship. This was because peppercorns were more valuable than gold and easily concealed in clothing.

FOLKLORE: In Eastern Europe, spilling pepper is very bad luck and is sure to cause an argument with your best friend. However, quickly sprinkling sugar onto the spilled pepper will resolve the problem.

FOLK MEDICINE: Second-century Greek physician Galen wrote: *"[black pepper] is strongly calefacient [warming] and desiccative [drying] thus very good for stomach problems"*.

An eye-watering remedy was given to an unfortunate patient suffering from colic: a mixture of honey boiled with pepper administered via the rectum. Unsurprisingly, Galen reports that this caused the patient *"extraordinary amounts of suffering"*, but once the treatment was stopped the patient made a full recovery.

In his ancient herbal, *De Materia Medica*, Greek physician Dioscorides prescribed black pepper as a treatment for pharyngitis and as a diuretic. He also advised that white pepper be applied topically for snake bites, eye diseases and in preparing an antidote for poison hemlock.

Animals in ancient Rome didn't escape the spicy qualities of black pepper either. To encourage mating, honey and pepper was rubbed on the hind quarters of female sheep. The burning sensation would prompt the ewe to find relief by rubbing herself on the nearest male.

OTHER COMMON USES: Black pepper essential oil is a calefacient, anti-inflammatory and antispasmodic, all of which can help ease the pain of tired muscles. Its warming effect improves blood circulation, which can also relieve the pain of arthritis.

Into 2 tbsp of carrier oil, add 5 drops of black pepper essential oil with 10 drops of ginger essential oil and mix well. This mixture can be rubbed onto sore and aching muscles.

Always do a patch test first.

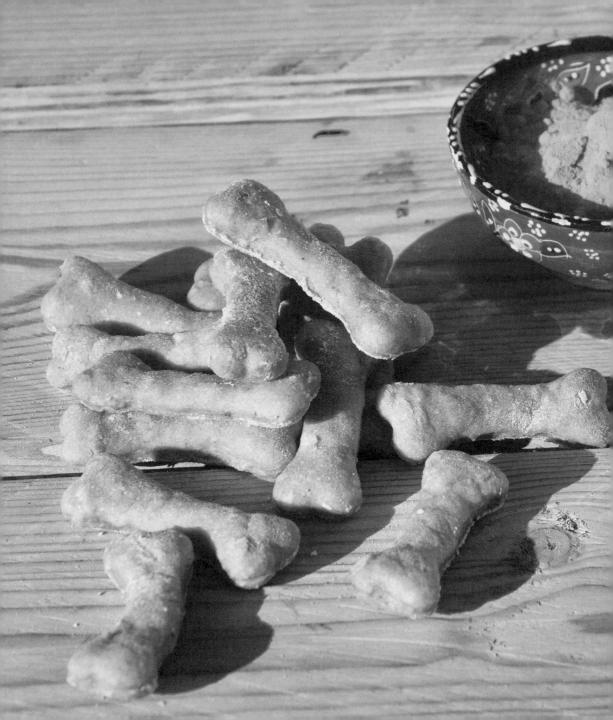

TURMERIC AND BLACK PEPPER DOG BISCUITS

Teaming black pepper with turmeric enhances the absorption of curcumin, the active ingredient in turmeric, making it even more effective as an anti-inflammatory.

When my elderly springer spaniel, Rosie, started to show signs of stiff joints, I wanted to give her something natural to help her. No matter how old your four-legged friend is, they will love these treats, and it might just do them some good, too.

Makes about 100 little bones for your best friend

INGREDIENTS

400 g wholemeal flour (I get this from my local flour mill)

1 large free-range egg, beaten

2 handfuls of porridge oats

6 tbsp vegetable oil or melted coconut oil

200 ml stock made with ½ a low-salt stock cube, cooled

1 tbsp turmeric powder

1 tsp ground black pepper

Equipment needed

Baking tray

Bone-shaped biscuit cutters

METHOD

Heat oven to 200°C (400°F).

Mix all the ingredients together to form a stiff dough. Add some water if necessary.

Dust a clean worktop with flour and roll out the dough to about ½ cm thick.

Cut out small shapes. Bone-shaped cutters are fun and available online.

Place the shapes on a baking tray dusted with flour.

Bake for 20–25 minutes or until the biscuits are golden brown and feel hard and dry.

Allow to cool completely on the tray.

Store in an airtight tin, where they will keep crunchy for a couple of months.

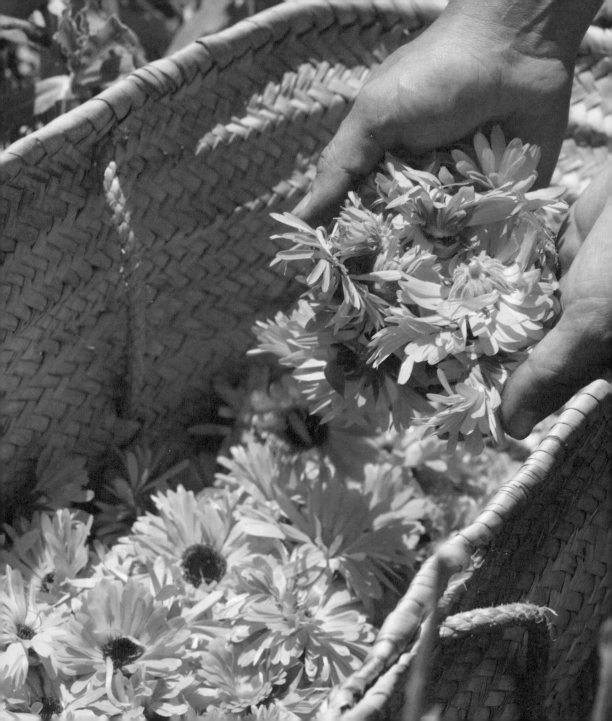

CALENDULA

Alternative names: Pot marigold, summer's bride, Mary gold, holigod, Jack on horseback, measle flower, drunkards

HOW TO IDENTIFY: This cheerful daisy-like flower comes in many shades, from pale creamy yellow to deep burnt orange. Calendula blooms from early spring well into autumn, producing many flower heads that can be dried for use in the medicine chest all year round.

HISTORY: Calendula was prized by the Ancient Greeks, Romans and Egyptians for its wonderful healing properties, as well as its use as a food colouring and to dye cloth.

Gertrude Jekyll, the renowned British horticulturalist, grew an abundance of calendula during the First World War to be sent to field hospitals in France. The cleansing and antiseptic properties of calendula were harnessed to speed up the healing of wounds.

Used by country folk to tell the time, calendula blossoms open up at around nine o'clock each morning and close again at three o'clock in the afternoon, signalling the end of the working day.

FOLKLORE: Hang a garland of calendula over the entrance of your home to remove all traces of witchcraft and prevent evil from entering your house.

Eating calendula petals will allow you to see the faery folk, and if you place them under your pillow, your dreams will surely come true.

Scatter calendula petals in your bathwater to give yourself a healthy, sunny glow guaranteed to draw admiring glances.

FOLK MEDICINE: A dozen calendula heads steeped in boiling water made a soothing "measle flower" tea that was traditionally given to children to ease the misery of measles.

Add a handful of calendula blossoms to your bath to soothe sunburned skin and ease the itch of insect bites and rashes.

OTHER COMMON USES: Calendula petals are edible, with a slightly peppery flavour, and can add a little sunshine to salads and cakes.

CALENDULA AND OAT SOOTHING FACE MASK

Calendula-infused oil calms, moisturizes, helps to reduce redness and promote skin health. Oats are anti-inflammatory and will gently exfoliate your skin, while honey's antibacterial properties will soothe acne and leave your skin glowing.

This recipe makes enough for one application; however, it's worth infusing extra calendula oil for other masks and skin care products.

INGREDIENTS

1 tbsp organic rolled oats

1 tbsp calendula-infused carrier oil (see page 14)

1 tbsp raw honey

Equipment needed

Pestle and mortar
or rolling pin

METHOD

Grind the oats a little with a pestle and mortar, or crush with the end of a rolling pin, leaving them just a little rough.

Combine the oats, oil and honey together in a small bowl.

Apply to the face and neck area; keep away from eyes.

Leave on for 15–20 minutes, then gently massage in small circles to exfoliate.

Rinse off with tepid water and gently pat dry.

Always do a patch test. Not to be used if pregnant, breastfeeding or if allergic to the daisy family.

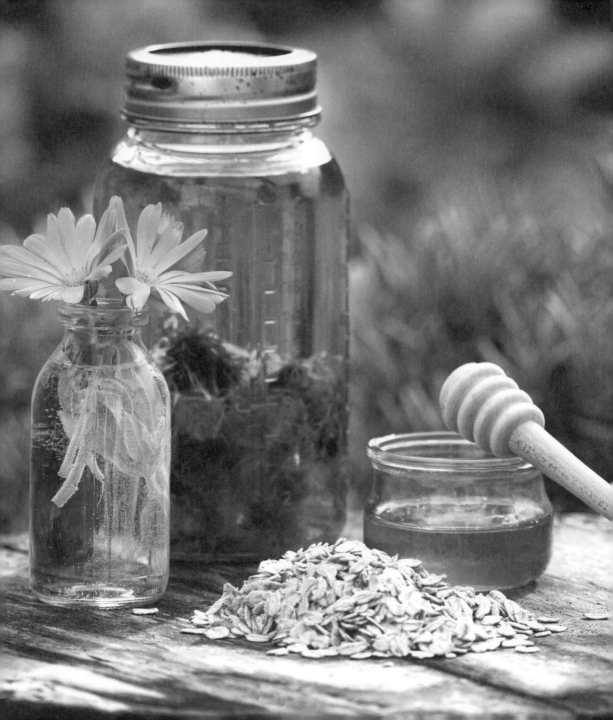

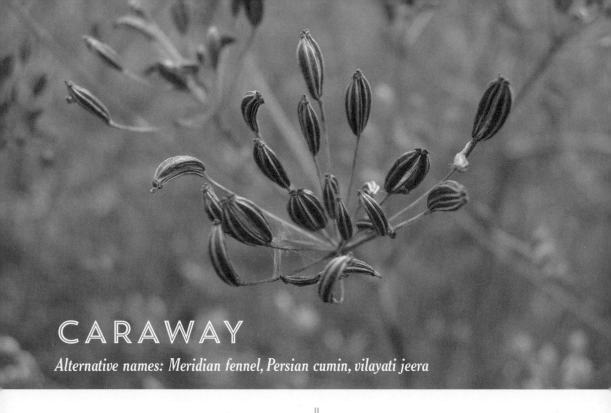

CARAWAY

Alternative names: Meridian fennel, Persian cumin, vilayati jeera

HOW TO IDENTIFY: Caraway is a member of the carrot family and has the same feathery leaves as its root vegetable cousin. Caraway seeds are actually fruits, which are smooth and crescent-shaped, with a distinctive scent and liquorice flavour.

HISTORY: The Ebers Papyrus is an Ancient Egyptian medical script of herbal knowledge containing recipes and remedies from 1550 BCE. It lists plants that were in common usage medicinally at the time, including mustard, garlic, coriander, mint, fennel, thyme, anise, wormwood and caraway.

The Romans brought caraway seeds to Britain, where the herb has grown happily ever since.

In the time of Elizabeth I, caraway "comfits", caraway seeds coated in sugar, were served after a meal to ease digestion, cleanse the palate and freshen breath. Caraway was popular enough to be mentioned in Shakespeare's play *Henry IV*, in a conversation between Justice Shallow and Falstaff:

"Nay, you shall see my orchard, where in an arbour we will eat last year's pippin of my own graffing, with a dish of caraways."

Caraway gradually fell out of favour on British tables until Queen Victoria married her German Prince Albert, when suddenly all things German became incredibly fashionable. Caraway is used in many German dishes, such as sauerkraut, sausages, rye bread and dumplings.

FOLKLORE: In Germany, it was believed that a plate of caraway seeds placed beneath a child's bed would protect them from witches, and a sprinkle of caraway seeds over a coffin would protect the dear departed from evil spirits.

There was a belief that any object containing caraway could not be stolen. This included people and animals who had eaten the seeds.

Chewing caraway seeds before kissing, apart from making your breath sweet, will also entice your partner to fall in love with you. Caraway thrown with rice at a wedding ensures love and fertility, and if you pop some in your spouse's food, they will always be faithful to you.

FOLK MEDICINE: Seeds ground into powder, mixed with vinegar and then made into a poultice will help heal bruises.

Blended with the crust of a freshly baked loaf, caraway was held to the ear as a traditional remedy for earache.

Sweetened caraway tea was given to infants with colic or trapped wind as a natural gripe water.

OTHER COMMON USES: If used in a diffuser, caraway essential oil can help combat the symptoms of a cold and is energizing and uplifting.

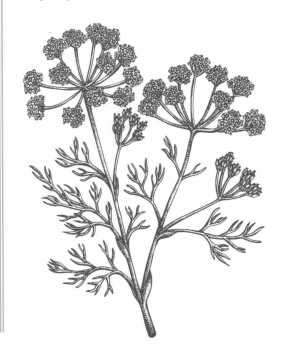

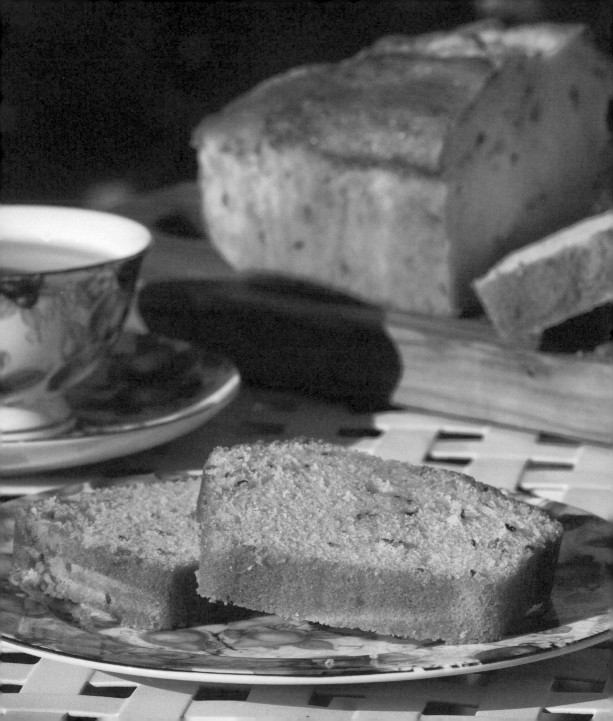

CARAWAY SEED CAKE

Caraway seed cake has been around since medieval times and was traditionally baked for agricultural workers after they had finished sowing the seed for that year. I'm guessing that, judging by the folklore, they were given caraway to ensure that they wouldn't leave the farm and work for anyone else.

The Victorians loved seed cake, but it is now often regarded as old fashioned and has since fallen out of favour. I think it's one tradition worth reviving.

INGREDIENTS

225 g plain flour

½ tsp baking powder

150 g softened butter

150 g caster sugar

3 large free-range eggs, beaten

2 tbsp milk

3 tsp caraway seeds

Equipment needed

1-kg loaf tin

METHOD

Preheat oven to 160°C (320°F)

Grease and line a 1-kg loaf tin.

Tip all ingredients into a bowl and beat until smooth.

Pour the mixture into the greased tin and level the surface.

Bake in the centre of the oven for about 50 minutes. At this point, insert a skewer into the centre of the cake – it should come out clean.

Leave to cool in the tin for 10 minutes, then transfer to a wire rack.

Put the kettle on.

Caraway seed shortbread is delicious, too. Use my recipe for autumn spice shortbread on page 137, substituting the autumn spice mix for 3 tsp of caraway seeds.

Caraway is best avoided if pregnant, breastfeeding or if you suffer from liver or gall bladder problems.

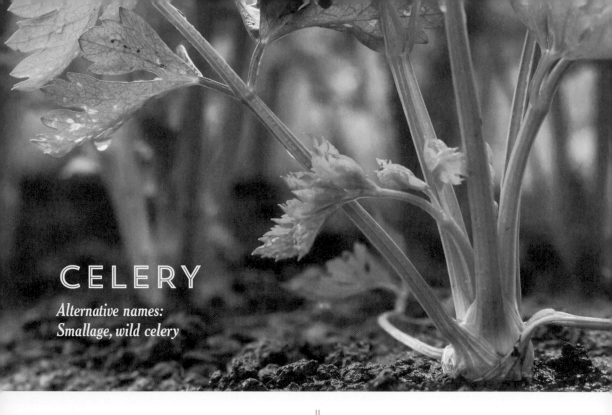

CELERY

Alternative names:
Smallage, wild celery

HOW TO IDENTIFY: Celery is a herbaceous plant of the parsley family with long pale green stringy stalks. Its leaves are very similar to parsley and have a distinctive smell.

HISTORY: "Smallage" is the wild variety of our cultivated celery, the difference being that the stems of wild celery are bitter and inedible. Native to the Middle East and the Mediterranean, wild celery was used as medicine in ancient China and as a flavouring by the Romans and Greeks.

Woven garlands of wild celery have also been found in early Ancient Egyptian tombs.

It wasn't until the late seventeenth century that a less bitter version of celery was widely cultivated and became a staple of European kitchens.

FOLKLORE: In northern Germany, celery was stuffed into the cracks of pigsties as protection from evil for all the animals inside.

Medieval recipes for love potions often included celery leaves for their purported aphrodisiac properties and the belief that they could increase virility.

Celery leaves, together with onion and garlic, can be hung in Greek doorways to bring good luck.

FOLK MEDICINE: In medieval medicine, "The Doctrine of Signatures" theory was posited on the logic that vegetables and flowers resembled the part of the body that they could heal. For example, walnuts were believed to be good for the brain whereas tomatoes have four chambers and could therefore heal the heart. Celery, meanwhile, is long like bones and stringy like hair, so it was believed to be beneficial for both healthy joints and bones as well as promoting lustrous locks.

In the seventeenth century, Culpeper wrote that celery seeds: *"disperse wind in the stomach and bowels. As this plant abounds in a pungent nitrous salt, it is therefore a detersive [detoxing substance] and diuretic."*

In the same century, English poet and writer Gervase Markham wrote *The English Housewife*, a text that instructed ladies on all the *"inward and outward virtues which ought to be in a complete woman"*. It gives a wonderful insight into the lives of contemporary women and what was expected of them. Markham's medical advice is particularly informative and occasionally a little disturbing. However, for sores that will not heal he sensibly recommends: *"take smallage [celery], groundsel, wild mallows and violet leaves; chop them small and boil them in milk with bruised oatmeal and sheep's suet, and so apply it to the sore."*

Witches are believed to eat celery seeds before flying away on their broomsticks, to prevent dizziness and improve their concentration in the air, while incense made using celery seeds and orris root is believed to increase psychic powers.

OTHER COMMON USES: An aromatic mirepoix (a mixture of sauteed vegetables) of celery, carrots and onions is the classic starting point for many savoury dishes.

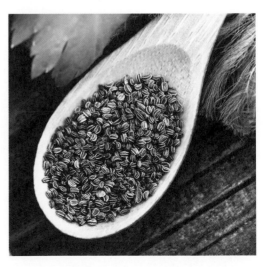

VEGETABLE BOUILLON POWDER

Shop-bought vegetable bouillon, although very convenient, may contain ingredients such as unsustainable palm oil and large amounts of salt. Making your own bouillon powder enables you to have total control over the ingredients you use, as well as meaning that you can add and remove elements to suit your own taste.

This recipe is plant based and gluten free. It can add that elusive "umami" flavour to any savoury dish or baking, making it a very handy addition to your pantry.

INGREDIENTS

120 g nutritional yeast (available from health food shops)

1 tsp celery seeds

1 tsp flaky sea salt

¼ tsp turmeric

1 tbsp Italian seasoning

1 tbsp garlic powder

1 tbsp thyme

1 tbsp parsley

1 tbsp onion powder

½ tsp ground black pepper

Equipment

Sterilized jar

METHOD

Place all the ingredients in a large bowl.

Give everything a really good mix – a whisk is handy for this.

Transfer the mixture into a clean airtight jar.

Store in a cool dark place and use within one year.

As a general rule, add 1 tbsp of store cupboard bouillon powder to 250 ml of hot water to make vegetable stock.

Celery and its seeds are allergens.

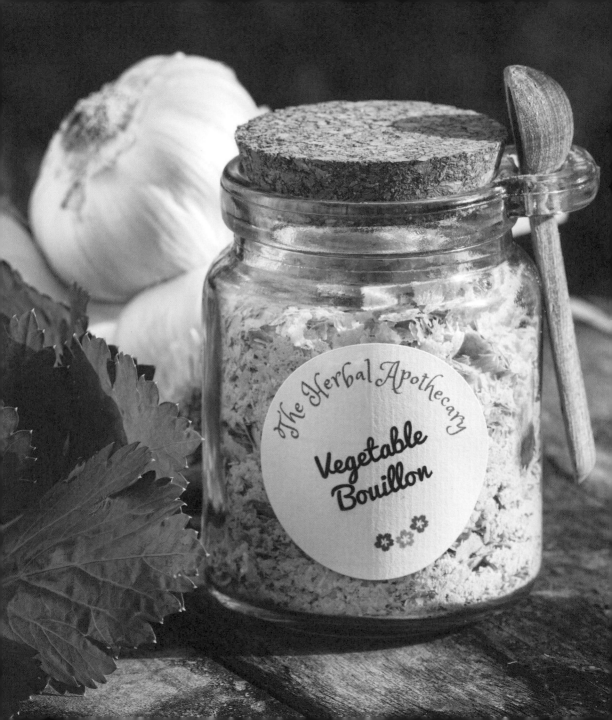

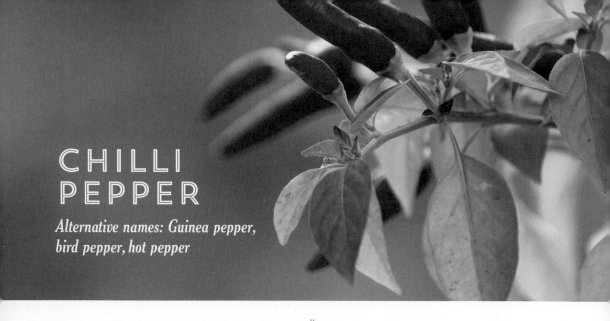

CHILLI PEPPER

Alternative names: Guinea pepper, bird pepper, hot pepper

HOW TO IDENTIFY: Chillies come in a huge variety of shapes, colours and degrees of heat. The Scoville scale is used to measure the "piquancy" of the pepper family. The number of Scovilles represents the amount of capsaicin present in the chilli pepper, a chemical irritant that makes chillies "hot". The Scoville scale starts with zero for a sweet bell pepper, goes to 250,000 for a scotch bonnet, and all the way up to 2.1 million for a California reaper!

HISTORY: Chillies were unheard of outside of the Caribbean and the Americas until Christopher Columbus encountered them in Hispaniola in the West Indies in 1492. He wrote: *"There is also plenty of agi, which is their pepper, which is more valuable than black pepper, and all the people eat nothing else, it being very wholesome."*

At the end of his second voyage in 1493, Columbus brought back chilli plants as gifts for the Spanish court. However, the King of Spain had tasked Columbus to bring back black pepper, which at the time was very expensive. As a result, the chillies weren't initially very well received.

Monks from Portugal and Spain are believed to have introduced chillies to Britain as both food and medicine in the sixteenth century.

FOLKLORE: Two large chilli peppers tied together with red ribbon can be placed under your pillow to prevent your partner from straying.

In some parts of southern Italy, chilli peppers are regarded as "the demon's spice". Strings of fresh chillies are hung over doorways or balconies to protect the occupants from the evil eye.

According to Hinduism, the goddess Alakshmi brings poverty, malice and deprivation into people's houses, unlike her twin sister Lakshmi, who brings wellness, love and prosperity. So naturally Lakshmi, who likes sweet things, is welcome to enter the home, but Alakshmi, who likes pungent and sour things, is not. A *"nimbu-mirchi"*, a talisman consisting of seven chillies and a lemon, is hung outside the door so that Alakshmi's appetite is satisfied before she enters the house, keeping her from crossing the threshold. At the same time, gifts of traditional sweet offerings such as phirni, halwa and laddoo are placed inside the home to entice Laksmi to enter.

FOLK MEDICINE: Culpeper knew chillies by the name of "Guinea peppers". He seems to have been quite a fan of their medicinal uses, but only once they had been *"corrected of their evil properties"* could they be *"of considerable service"*. He writes that:

"A little pulpy part of the fruit, held in the mouth, cures the tooth-ache; and if bruised and applied externally to the part affected [...] it is good for the quinsey [an abscess on the tonsils]."

In the West Indies, chilli oil was rubbed into the scalp to stimulate hair growth. In Mexico and Latin America, chilli powder was rubbed onto children's thumbs as a deterrent to thumb sucking. Meanwhile, naughty or lazy children in the Andes were made to inhale the smoke from burning chilli seeds to make them sneeze and become obedient.

On a lighter note, chillies were used as a cure for flatulence and rubbed onto painful arthritic joints. If you try this remedy, be careful not to use very hot chillies because they will literally burn your skin!

OTHER COMMON USES: Chillies are versatile and can be included in both savoury and sweet dishes – I'm a big fan of chilli chocolate!

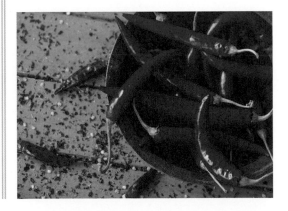

IMMUNITY-BOOSTING CHILLI TEA

Chillies contain capsaicin, which can help relieve congestion and is also a useful natural antibiotic. Ginger has antioxidant, antiviral, antibacterial and anti-inflammatory properties; garlic helps to boost the immune system; lemons are high in both vitamin C and antioxidants; and honey is soothing as well as being antibacterial. These ingredients and their therapeutic properties add up to the perfect remedy for colds and flu.

Serves two

INGREDIENTS

½ a fresh chilli, chopped (be careful, these can vary in heat, so always check the labelling)

3 cloves of organic garlic, peeled and crushed

3 tbsp organic ginger, grated

500 ml boiled water

Juice and grated rind of 1 organic lemon

Raw honey to sweeten to taste

Equipment needed

Teapot or heatproof jug

METHOD

Put the chilli, garlic and ginger into a teapot or heatproof jug.

Pour the boiled water over the ingredients. Cover the container and leave to steep for at least 10 minutes.

Add the lemon juice, lemon rind and honey.

Strain the mixture into a cup, then snuggle up and enjoy.

Aim to drink at least two cups of chilli tea a day to reap the full benefit of its healing properties.

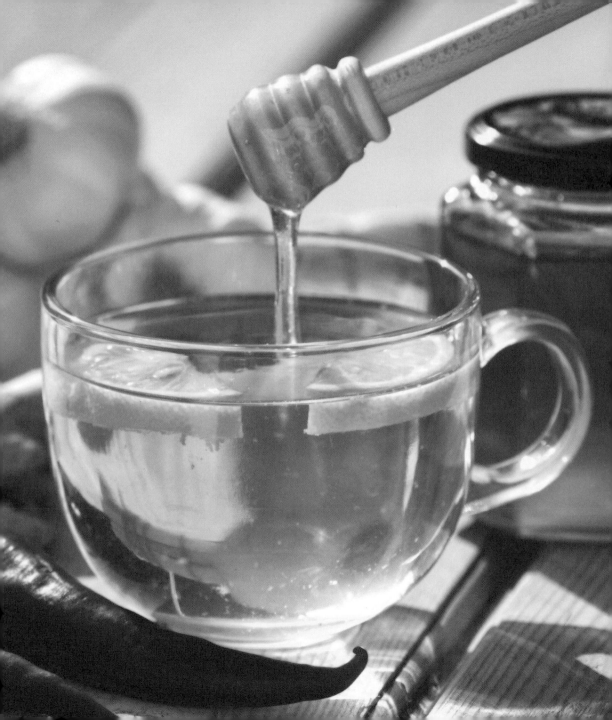

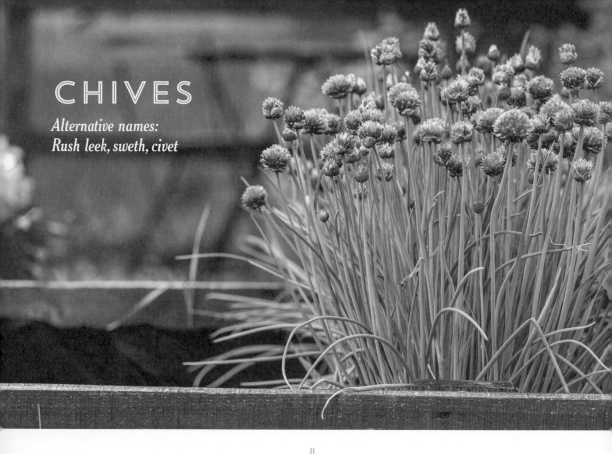

CHIVES

Alternative names:
Rush leek, sweth, civet

HOW TO IDENTIFY: Chives are closely related to the onion family in both taste and smell. Their long, slender leaves are topped with a purple pom-pom flower throughout summer.

HISTORY: Chives, which have been used as both medicine and food by the Chinese for well over 5,000 years, were brought to European shores by the Romans. Chives and other herbs still grow in the crevices of Hadrian's Wall in northern England, where they were originally planted for use by Roman physicians.

Chives weren't cultivated in Britain until the medieval period, when they were used to discourage insects or else as a decorative plant.

In the sixteenth century, Scottish surgeons would regularly forage for chives and other herbs in early summer at Hadrian's Wall to replenish their apothecary stores.

FOLKLORE: The Romani people believed that hanging bunches of dried chives around the home would ward off disease and evil spirits.

Gather 13 stalks of chive on Tuesday, tie them together with cotton string and hang them in the home to dispel negative energy.

Chives can also be used in fortune telling; if you throw the chives into the air while thinking of a question, the answer can be interpreted from the way the chives fall onto the ground.

It was believed that a bundle of chives hung over a child's bed would keep the room free from sickness.

FOLK MEDICINE: The Romans had multiple uses for chives, including as a treatment for sunburn and sore throats, to increase blood pressure, as a diuretic and even to help stop bleeding.

Culpeper didn't have a very high opinion of chives at all: *"If they be eaten raw, they send up very hurtful vapours to the brain, causing troublesome sleep, and spoiling the eyesight."*

Juice from the leaves can be used to treat fungal infections, eradicate mildew, strengthen hair and nails and even as an aphrodisiac – although the Roman poet Marcus Valerius Martialis noted that:

"He who bears chives on his breath, is safe from being kissed to death."

OTHER COMMON USES: Chives are great companion plants for roses because they repel both Japanese beetles and the fungal disease black spot. Similarly, when planted near apple trees they help to keep the airborne fungus that causes apple scab at bay.

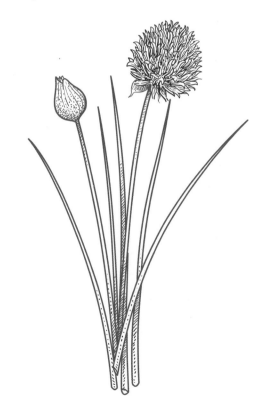

CHIVE PESTO

Raw chives add a real twist to this favourite family recipe. I like to keep a little basil in the mix because I love the flavour – you could use all chives if you wish.

Serves two

INGREDIENTS

15 g washed and roughly chopped chives

10 g fresh basil

2 cloves of garlic, crushed

A handful of walnuts, pine nuts or almonds

6 tbsp olive oil

30 g grated parmesan or plant-based alternative

Salt and pepper to season

Equipment needed

Stick blender or food processor

METHOD

Pulse the chives, basil and garlic in a blender until mixed.

Add the walnuts and pulse again.

Pour in the olive oil and the grated cheese, then pulse until the texture is to your taste.

Season with salt and pepper.

Stir through freshly cooked pasta.

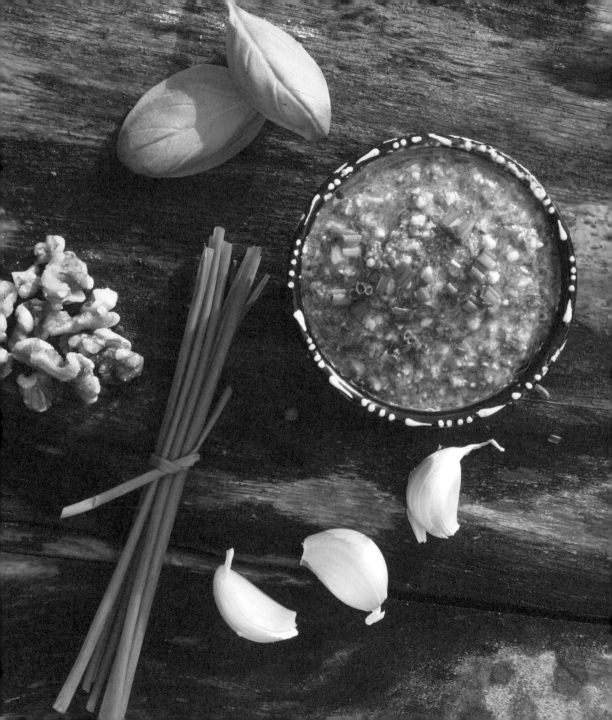

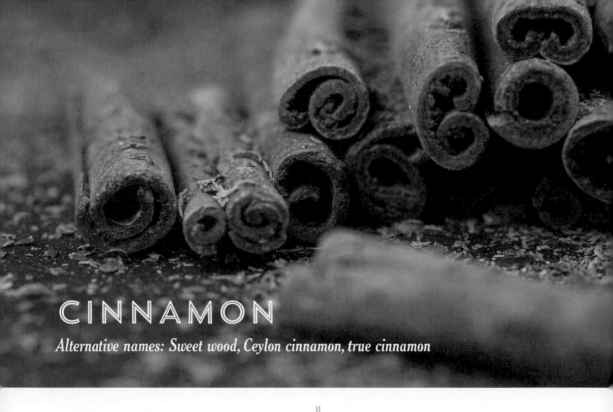

CINNAMON

Alternative names: Sweet wood, Ceylon cinnamon, true cinnamon

HOW TO IDENTIFY: Cinnamon is the aromatic inner bark of a bushy evergreen shrub native to India and Sri Lanka. The inner bark is stripped from the outer layer, naturally forming quill shapes or curls as it dries.

HISTORY: In the first century CE, cinnamon was incredibly valuable. In fact, Pliny the Elder recorded that just 350 g of cinnamon was worth the same amount as 5 kg of silver. Cinnamon was also considered sacred, and every Roman emperor kept a supply of it in his treasury. Nero, who murdered his wife Poppaea Sabina while she was pregnant, gave her the most lavish funeral pyre built from all the cinnamon in Rome as a public show of remorse.

The Ancient Egyptians used cinnamon essential oil along with cassia and myrrh in the mummification process. Similarly, the Hebrews also used it as an ingredient in their holy anointing oils.

Sri Lanka, which was the largest producer of cinnamon at the time, came under the control of the Portuguese in the sixteenth century. They established a fort on the island, just to protect their control of this valuable spice. The Dutch, however, seized control of the island in the seventeenth century, destroying all other cinnamon plantations to ensure that they kept their monopoly – and therefore the highest price.

Plague doctors in seventeenth-century Europe wore quite frightening protective clothing in an attempt to keep themselves safe from the disease. A long black waxed coat, wide-brimmed hat and gloves were topped off with a bird-like mask filled with a mixture of 55 herbs and spices such as cinnamon, lavender, camphor and juniper berries. Plague doctors believed the herbs and spices would keep away the evil airborne miasmas that they maintained caused the plague.

By 1833, places such as Borneo, Mauritius and Guyana found that they were able to grow cinnamon quite easily. This caused the price of the herb to drop universally and cinnamon became far more accessible.

FOLKLORE: One ritual involves blowing cinnamon powder across your front door on the first day of every month. This is said to improve the energy in your home and invite prosperity, happiness and abundance across the threshold.

FOLK MEDICINE: Historically, cinnamon was believed to cure everything from kidney problems and the common cold to freckles and even snakebites.

In Chinese medicine, cinnamon is administered to promote a youthful appearance and improve complexion and also as a treatment for menstrual cramps. It is sometimes used as a natural painkiller, to combat bad breath, improve memory and as an aphrodisiac.

Medieval physicians used cinnamon to treat coughs, hoarseness and sore throats.

Gervase Markham told his seventeenth-century housewives to use cinnamon to ease any sharp stabbing pain just below the ribs experienced after exercise: *"Take a good store of cinnamon grated and put it in a posset ale very hot and drink it, and it is a present cure."*

In *A Modern Herbal* (1931), president of the British Guild of Herb Growers Maud Grieve wrote that cinnamon *"stops vomiting, relieves flatulence and given with chalk and astringents is useful for diarrhoea and haemorrhage of the womb"*.

OTHER COMMON USES: Mulled apple juice simmered with cinnamon sticks, oranges, ginger, cloves, nutmeg and cardamom is an aromatic Christmas favourite.

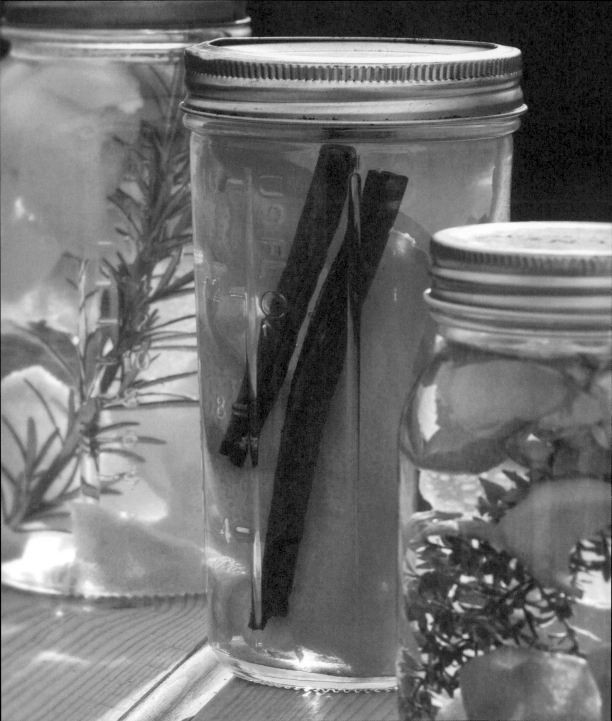

CINNAMON AND ORANGE CLEANING SPRAY

Cinnamon has antibacterial, antiviral and antifungal properties. Combine this with white vinegar's ability to dissolve grime and mineral deposits as well as the natural antibacterial properties of citrus fruit, and we can make a powerful eco-friendly all-purpose cleaning product very cheaply and easily.

INGREDIENTS

1 litre white vinegar

Enough orange peel to fill a 1-litre jar

2 cinnamon sticks

Equipment needed

1-litre jar

Alternative vinegar ideas:

Lime peels and thyme
Lemon peels and rosemary

METHOD

Half fill your jar with vinegar.

Save the peel (without the pith) from some oranges and pop it in with the vinegar.

Once your jar is filled with peel, top it up with vinegar and add two cinnamon sticks.

Seal the jar with a non-metallic lid, or top with some cling film and an elastic band.

Leave the mixture for at least three weeks.

Strain into a jug and dilute 1:1 with water. Add less water for a stronger cleaner.

Spray onto surfaces, allow to sit for a minute or two and then wipe off.

Avoid using vinegar-based cleaner on natural stone surfaces or hardwood floors.

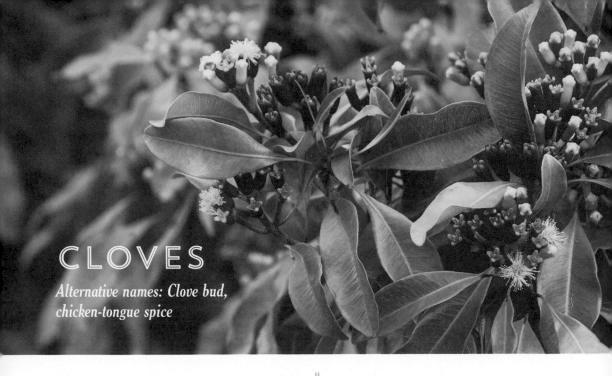

CLOVES

Alternative names: Clove bud, chicken-tongue spice

HOW TO IDENTIFY: Primarily grown in Madagascar and Indonesia, cloves are dried, unopened buds from the evergreen tree *Syzygium aromaticum*. Cloves get their name from "*clavus*" the Latin word for "nails", referring to their similarity to metal nails.

HISTORY: Cloves are one of the earliest spices to be written about in Asian literature. Records from the Chinese Han dynasty of the second century BCE document how cloves were chewed to freshen breath as well as being used in medicine and food.

The trade in cloves gradually spread to Greece and Egypt. Merchants then imported them into Europe to be used to preserve, flavour and garnish food.

The spice trade was controlled initially by the Chinese, then the Portuguese and finally the Dutch, who destroyed any tree outside their territory to ensure that cloves were worth their weight in gold.

FOLKLORE: Cloves can be burned to cleanse a property, attracting both wealth and good luck, with the added bonus of stopping any malicious gossip, too.

Carrying or wearing cloves will make you more attractive and keep your friendships strong.

Cloves buried among rice will keep away insects.

Sucking two whole cloves will disperse any desire that you have to overindulge in alcohol and could perk up your love life.

FOLK MEDICINE: In the medieval period, those that could afford them would place cloves in their gums to numb the pain of toothache. Although this remedy was very effective for temporary relief, if cloves are left in the gums for a prolonged period of time they can kill the nerves, resulting in tooth loss!

The sixteenth-century British herbalist John Gerard tells us that the oil from cloves *"when dropped in the eyes sharpens sight and cleans away any cloud or web. If four drams of clove powder is mixed with milk and drunk, this will result in the act of generation [pregnancy]."*

In the following century, Culpeper comments that *"cloves improve digestion, stop looseness [of the bowels], provoke lust and quicken the eyesight".*

OTHER COMMON USES: Cloves, along with cinnamon, ginger and allspice, are commonly used to create wonderful baking at Christmas time, with whole cloves being pushed into oranges to make fragrant festive pomanders.

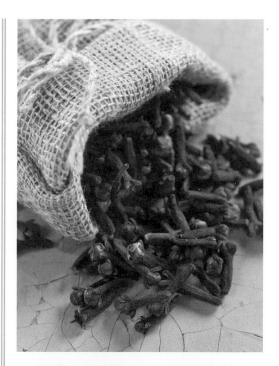

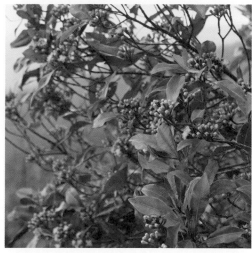

NATURAL VAPOUR RUB

Cloves are one of the powerhouses of natural medicine, with anti-inflammatory, antibacterial, antimicrobial, analgesic and anaesthetic properties. Many dental products contain clove oil, and you might recognize the distinctive aroma from your visits to the dentist.

This recipe makes a handy decongestant oil with all the benefits of vapour rub but without the sustainability implications of the petroleum industry.

INGREDIENTS

125 ml carrier oil

10 drops clove essential oil

10 drops lemon
essential oil

10 drops peppermint
essential oil

10 drops eucalyptus
essential oil

Equipment needed

Sterilized airtight glass
bottle with stopper

METHOD

Combine all the ingredients together in a glass airtight bottle.

Stopper, and shake well before use.

To ease a night-time cough, rub generously onto the soles of the feet then cover with socks. Alternatively, rub on the chest to help ease congestion.

Use within one year.

For a solid rub, melt 15 g of beeswax gently into the oil before adding the essential oils and pour into a shallow container to set.

Always do a patch test. Not recommended for use on children under 12.

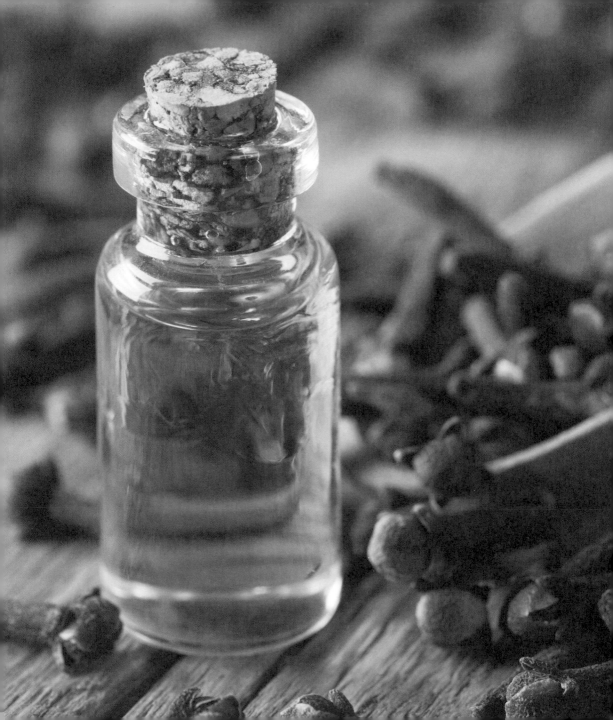

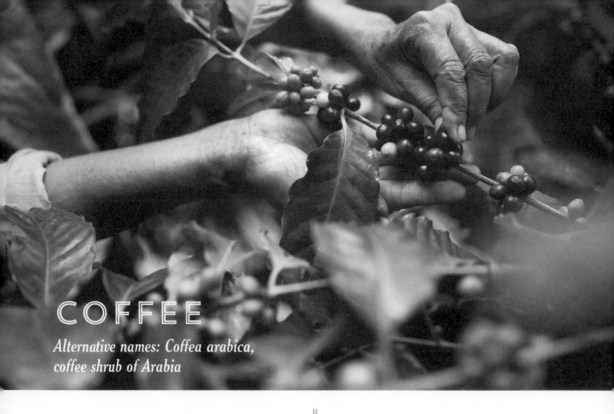

COFFEE

Alternative names: Coffea arabica, coffee shrub of Arabia

HOW TO IDENTIFY: The arabica coffee plant has evergreen shiny leaves, sweetly scented white flowers and red fruit. Each fruit produces two green seeds which, once roasted, become coffee beans.

HISTORY: Legend tells us that centuries ago a young Ethiopian goat-herder named Kaldi noticed that his goats became particularly energetic after they had eaten the berries from a certain tree. Kaldi reported this to the abbot of the local monastery who, on making a drink from the same berries, discovered that he could stay awake even during the long hours of evening prayer. Soon all the monks were consuming this energizing drink and word began to spread far and wide.

Opinion on how coffee beans ended up being roasted is divided. Some think that the tradition began in Saudi Arabia when coffee branches were burned over a fire to roast the beans. Others believe that the seeds were roasted with ginger and cinnamon in the Yemen to make a drink called *"qishr"*, long before the widespread use of coffee.

Travellers returning from the Middle East told tales of "an unusual dark black beverage" and by the seventeenth century coffee had made its way to Britain and most of Europe.

At first, coffee was regarded by the clergy as "the bitter invention of Satan". It wasn't until Pope Clement VIII tried it in 1615, and finding it most satisfying, granted it papal approval, that it began to gain popularity.

FOLKLORE: According to Ancient Ethiopian folklore, the god Waqa was so upset at having to sentence one of his most loyal men to death that coffee beans sprouted from the tears running down his face. The legend states that while other plants may grow easily, coffee beans will only germinate if they are watered by the tears of a god.

An eye mask filled with coffee beans will prevent nightmares and coffee grounds can be read in exactly the same way as tea leaves in a form of divination. Washing your floors with an infusion of coffee is believed to keep ghosts away.

FOLK MEDICINE: Although the Pope clearly liked coffee as a beverage, Culpeper clearly did not. Nor did he recognize any therapeutic benefit. He described coffee as: *"insipid, having neither scent nor taste, but being pounded and baked, as they do prepare it to make coffee-liquor with it then stinks loathsomely [...] they also say it makes them sober when they are drunk... or at least think themselves so".*

In 1652, "men only" coffee houses were on the rise in the St Paul's area of London. Culpeper died in 1654, so it is unlikely that he ever knew how unpopular his opinion of coffee would turn out to be!

Coffee is used in traditional Chinese medicine for the treatment of fever, irregular heartbeat, asthma and chronic diarrhoea.

OTHER COMMON USES: Coffee grounds are used by gardeners to deter slugs and snails from feasting on their crops. When composted, this waste product can add essential potassium and phosphates to the soil.

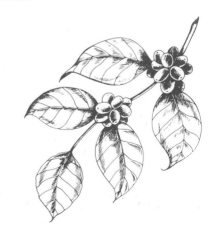

COFFEE BODY SCRUB

If you are a regular customer, many coffee shops will happily give you a bag of used grounds for free – especially if you make them some of this delightful scrub in exchange. This is not only a perfect gift for family and friends, but also a great way to reuse a waste product that would otherwise end up in landfill.

Many cosmetics use extracts from the coffee berry because it is rich in caffeine and other antioxidants, both of which are known to be beneficial to skin and hair. This coffee scrub recipe will gently exfoliate your skin, while Epsom salts will help soothe irritation. Rosemary essential oil will stimulate circulation, lavender essential oil will calm sensitive skin and tea tree oil is an anti-inflammatory.

You can adapt the recipe to your own needs and scent preferences, adding more carrier oil if you prefer a looser scrub.

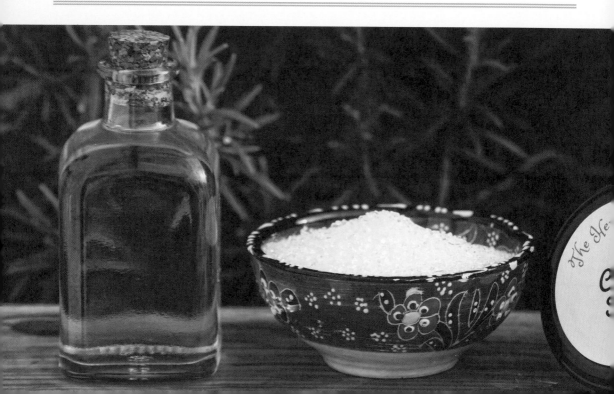

INGREDIENTS

50 g coffee grounds

50 g Epsom salts or fine sea salt

3 tbsp carrier oil (olive oil
or sunflower oil is fine)

10 drops lavender essential oil

10 drops tea tree essential oil

5 drops rosemary essential oil

Equipment needed

Sterilized glass jar

METHOD

Combine all the ingredients together.

Transfer into a glass jar and seal well.

Apply a generous scoop to the body using circular movements. Leave for 1 minute to give the oils time to work their moisturizing magic on your skin.

Rinse off with warm water.

Pat dry.

Always do a patch test. Not recommended for use on the face.

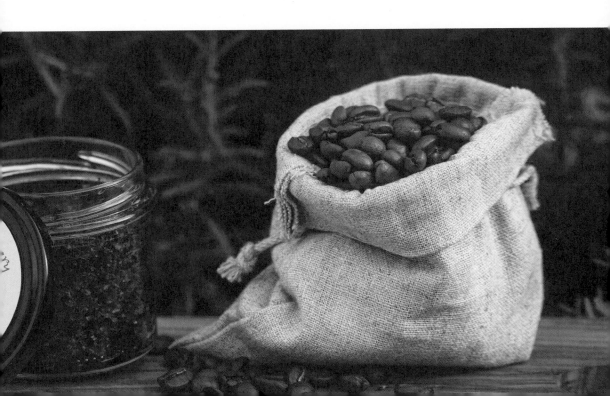

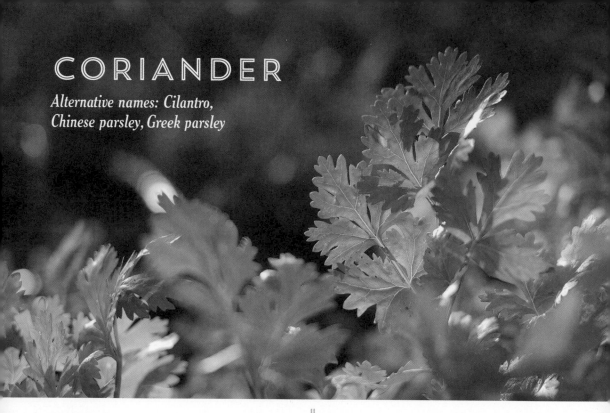

CORIANDER

Alternative names: Cilantro,
Chinese parsley, Greek parsley

HOW TO IDENTIFY: Coriander is an annual herb with feathery aromatic leaves. It is very similar in appearance to parsley but has a fresh, earthy smell. Coriander is both a herb and a spice. The leaves are a herb sometimes referred to as cilantro and the seeds are the spice, coriander.

HISTORY: Coriander was common in the Nile region of Africa; seeds were placed in the tomb of the boy king Tutankhamun to protect him on his final journey and ensure rebirth in the Otherworld. Ancient Egyptians also infused coriander into wine and used it in many of their culinary recipes, as well as adding it to hot baths to ease fevers.

Later, coriander was referenced in the Bible: *"The people of Israel called the bread manna. It was white like coriander seed..."* (Exodus 16:31)

For a long time, coriander was thought to have arrived in Britain via the Roman invaders. However, seeds imported from the Mediterranean have since been found in Bronze Age excavations, dating their arrival as much earlier.

Coriander comfits, seeds coated in sugar, were offered to guests after their meal at medieval banquets to aid digestion and prevent embarrassing wind and bloating.

The British love affair with spicy food has been around a lot longer than you may think. In 1931, Maud Grieve published her recipe for Lucknow curry powder, using coriander: *"1 oz. ginger, 1 oz. coriander seed, 1 oz. cardamom seed, ¼ oz. best cayenne powder, 3 oz. turmeric. Have the best ingredients powdered at the druggists into a fine powder and sent home in different papers. Mix them well before the fire, then put the mixture into a wide-mouthed bottle. Cork well, and keep it in a dry place."*

FOLKLORE: Coriander was added to love potions during the medieval and Renaissance periods because it was believed to have powerful aphrodisiac properties. Robert Turner, the seventeenth-century astrologer and herbalist, seems to agree, writing that coriander consumed with wine *"stimulates the animal passions"*.

It was believed that coriander grown in the garden would protect the gardener and all their household. Harvest a bunch of the herb and hang it inside the house for extra protection.

The participants at Pagan handfasting ceremonies sometimes drank wine infused with coriander to ensure fertility. Coriander seeds can also be thrown instead of confetti at weddings and handfastings.

Pregnant women were encouraged to eat coriander if they wished their child to be a genius.

FOLK MEDICINE: Pliny the Elder pronounced that *"the best coriander, as is generally agreed, is the Egyptian"*, for healing sores, eradicating intestinal parasites and relieving cholera.

A traditional home remedy for conjunctivitis is to bathe the closed eyelids with coriander-seed tea.

Traditional Chinese medicine recommends coriander to soothe toothache, nausea, piles and measles.

OTHER COMMON USES: A rinse made from coriander-leaf tea will promote fuller hair growth.

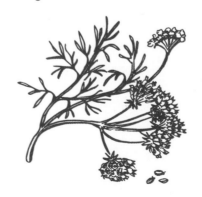

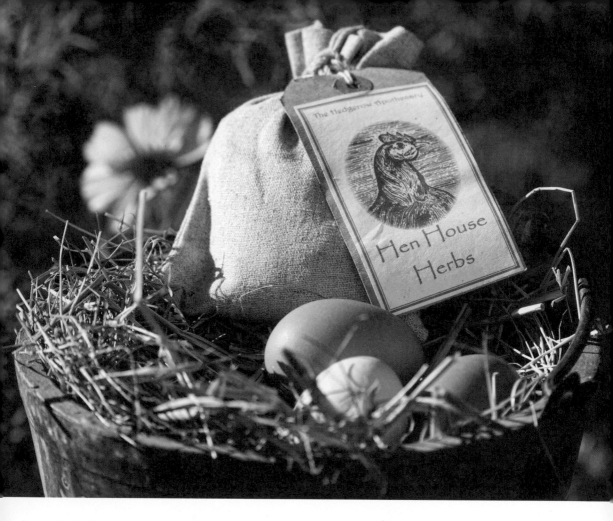

HEN HOUSE HERBS

Herbs are not only beneficial for our own health but also the well-being of the animals that depend on us. Even if you don't keep chickens yourself, these herb mixes are perfect gifts for friends who do. If you're lucky, you might get some eggs in exchange. Pick and choose the dried herbs with benefits that suit the needs of your flock.

Choose equal quantities of any of the following dried herbs:

BASIL: Antibacterial. Supports mucous membrane health.

CALENDULA: Antioxidant and insect repellent. Good for feet and beaks. Good for vibrant egg yolks.

CORIANDER: Antioxidant and fungicide. High in vitamin A for vision and vitamin K for blood clotting. Builds strong bones.

LAVENDER: Insecticidal stress reliever.

OREGANO: Natural antibiotic. Protects against avian flu, E. coli and infectious bronchitis.

PARSLEY: Laying stimulant with multiple health benefits. High in vitamins A, B and D, calcium, iron, magnesium, selenium and zinc.

ROSEMARY: Pain relief and insecticide. Supports respiratory health.

SAGE: Antioxidant and anti-parasitic. Helps to combat salmonella in the eggs. Laying stimulant.

THYME: Antibacterial, antioxidant and antiparasitic. Supports respiratory health.

YARROW: Antibacterial and anti-inflammatory. Clears sinuses and respiratory systems.

METHOD

Mix your chosen herbs together.

Store in an airtight container.

Mix a few Hen House Herbs with your chickens' normal food and sprinkle some into the nest box, too.

Any of the herbs listed above would also be beneficial growing around the chicken coop so your flock can forage at will.

Coriander is an allergen.

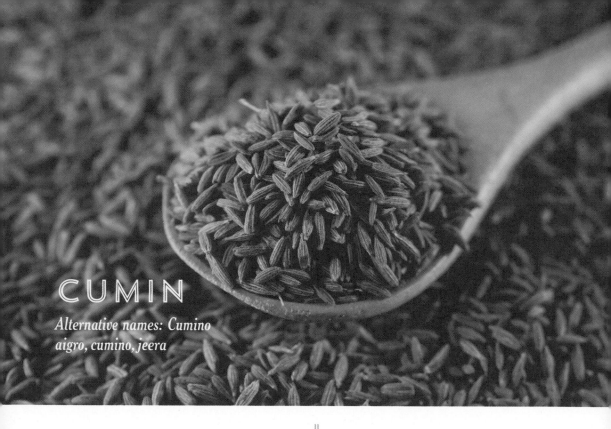

CUMIN

Alternative names: Cumino aigro, cumino, jeera

HOW TO IDENTIFY: The cumin plant is an annual herbaceous herb with slender branched stems and lace-like flowers, growing to about 30–60 cm (1–2 feet). Cumin seeds are ready to harvest, usually by hand, when the seeds become dry and brittle.

HISTORY: Ancient Egyptians used cumin as part of the mummification process. It was regarded as the "king of condiments" by the Ancient Greeks and Romans, who kept cumin as a cheaper substitute for black pepper, which was very expensive, in its own special container alongside salt.

Cumin is even mentioned in the Bible: *"You give a tenth of your spices – mint, dill and cumin. But you have neglected the more important matters of the law – justice, mercy and faithfulness."* (Matthew 23:23)

Cumin originated in Western Asia, where it has been cultivated since ancient times. Today, India and Iran are the main producers of cumin worldwide. It is also grown in Argentina, Morocco, Ukraine, Egypt, Lebanon,

Malta, Mexico, Afghanistan, Pakistan, Turkey, Central America and Central Asia.

FOLKLORE: Jeelakarra Bellam is an important part of Telugu Hindu wedding rituals. Cumin (which is bitter) is mixed into a paste with a type of sugar called jaggery (which is sweet) and exchanged by the couple to signify that they will stick together through the bitter and sweet challenges of their lives. The paste is wrapped in a betel leaf and the couple feed each other while the priest reads the Hindu Vedas (sacred scriptures).

Elsewhere, a happy life awaits the bride and groom who carry cumin seeds or flowers during their wedding ceremony.

Folklore tells us that cumin, just like caraway, has "the gift of retention", which applies to both people and objects. Burglars attempting to steal anything containing cumin from the home would be trapped inside the house. Wives should give their husbands bread or wine seasoned with cumin to keep them faithful, and a little cumin added to bird food prevents racing pigeons from straying too far.

FOLK MEDICINE: British herbalist John Gerard wrote of cumin seeds that they: *"scattereth and breaketh all the windiness of the stomache, belly, guts and matrix [uterus]; prepared as broth cumin seeds are good for the chest and cold lungs; when mixed with vinegar and smelled, will stop nosebleeds".*

One seventeenth-century cure for sore eyes recommends: *"Take a gallon or two of the dregs of strong ale, and put thereto a handful of cumin, and as much salt, and then distil in a limbeck and the water is most precious to wash the eyes with."*

Cumin mixed with salt can be rubbed into sore gums to reduce the swelling and a gargle is useful to soothe mouth ulcers.

Unani medicine is an alternative medicine method that originated in ancient Greece, now mainly practised in India, which uses cumin to treat insomnia, fever, haemorrhoids, diarrhoea and even scorpion stings.

OTHER COMMON USES: This warm, aromatic spice is one of the main components of garam masala. Cumin is traditionally added to curries, Mexican dishes such as chilli con carne and is used as a rub in North African lamb dishes.

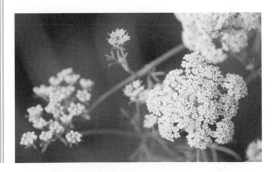

JEERA WATER

Due to its high content of iron, manganese, calcium, vitamin B1 and phosphorus, cumin is believed to promote *"agni"* (from the Sanskrit meaning "digestive fire"). Agni helps to stimulate digestion and relieve bloating. As a result, jeera water is traditionally taken first thing in the morning to kick-start your digestion for the day.

Serves two

INGREDIENTS

1 tsp organic cumin seeds, lightly crushed

500 ml filtered water

Raw honey (optional)

Squeeze of lemon juice (optional)

Equipment needed

Stainless-steel pan

Sieve

METHOD

Gently dry roast the cumin seeds in a stainless-steel pan until the aroma is released.

Add the water to the pan and bring to the boil.

Pop on a lid and simmer for 10 minutes.

Take off the heat and allow to cool to room temperature or lukewarm.

Strain out the cumin seeds, sweeten with honey and add a squeeze of lemon to taste.

Use cumin with caution if you are allergic to the umbellifer family of plants.

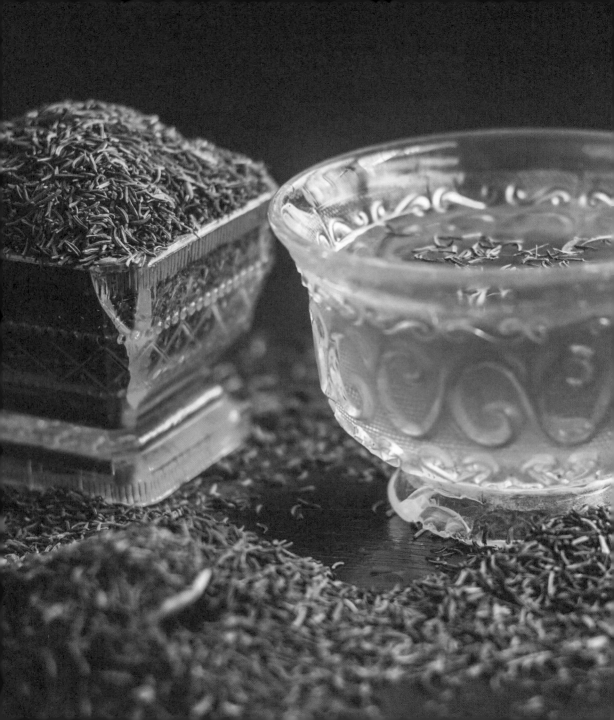

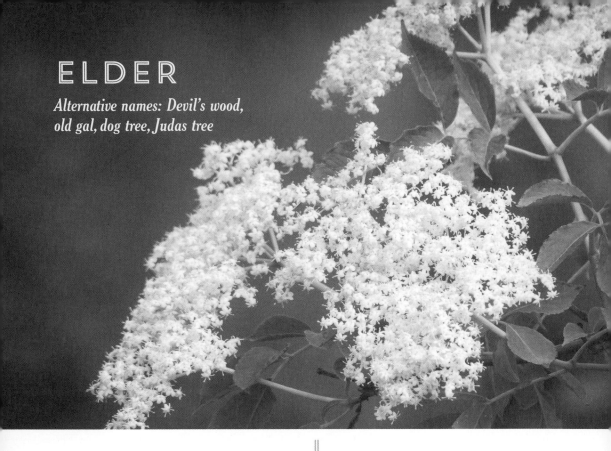

ELDER

Alternative names: Devil's wood, old gal, dog tree, Judas tree

HOW TO IDENTIFY: Common in European hedgerows and woods, this large shrub has a corky bark that splits as it matures. The leaves comprise five to seven oval leaflets with feathery edges. Clusters of creamy white fragrant flowers appear in early summer followed by small dark purple berries in early autumn, which are edible once cooked.

HISTORY: The hollow stems were used by blacksmiths to blow air onto their forge fires and children once enjoyed using them as peashooters.

Elder leaves have insect-repelling properties and were hung from horses' bridles to keep flies away.

FOLKLORE: If you happen to be underneath an elder tree on Midsummer's Night, you may be serenaded by the faery folk playing whistles and pipes made from the hollow stems of the elder tree.

An elder tree that has seeded itself in your garden is said to prevent evil spirits, negative influences and lightning from striking your home. One planted by your cowshed will protect your cattle.

Elders were believed to be inhabited by witches who had transformed themselves into the tree to escape capture. You must always seek permission from the resident witch before you forage from her tree or suffer the consequences.

According to the Wiccan Rede, a twentieth-century moral guide for wiccans (modern Pagans) to abide by:

*"Elder is the lady's tree,
Burn it not or cursed
you'll be."*

FOLK MEDICINE: The elder is known by country folk as "nature's medicine chest"; every part of this wonderful tree can be turned into a remedy.

Toothache caused by evil spirits could be cured by chewing on a twig, which was then left on top of a boundary wall while saying: "Depart thou evil spirit."

Culpeper also recommended elder for toothache: *"Take the inner rind of an elder tree, and bruise it, and put thereto a little pepper, and make it into balls, and hold them between the teeth that ache."*

Warts could be transferred onto the elder by cutting the same number of notches as you had warts into a piece of root or twig, rubbing it on your warts and then burying it. As the elder decomposed, your warts would vanish.

In his seventeenth-century book *The English Housewife*, Markham writes: *"To make a poultice to cure any ague sore take elder leaves and seethe them in milk till they be soft, then take them up and strain them; and then boil again till it be thick, and so use it to the sore as occasion shall serve."*

Scalds and burns were treated with elder flowers mixed with lard to make an ointment. The flowers can also be infused with honey to make a tea to soothe the symptoms of hay fever.

The berries are full of antioxidants and vitamin C and were, and still are, used to make an effective home remedy for coughs, colds and sore throats.

OTHER COMMON USES: An English summer wouldn't be the same without a fragrant glass of elderflower cordial in the sunshine. The cordial can also be drizzled over cakes and pancakes and makes a gin and tonic very special indeed!

ELDER LEAF SALVE

A salve made from infused elder leaves applied topically helps to heal bruises and chilblains, soothes aching muscles and acts as a natural insect repellent. Gather young leaves on a dry day from an elder that is away from pollution, using a field guide to help you to identify the shrub correctly. This easy-to-make salve will be a useful addition to your herbal apothecary.

Makes approx. 225 ml

INGREDIENTS

A handful of elder leaves

200 ml carrier oil

25 g natural beeswax

20 drops lavender or rosemary essential oil

Equipment needed

Piece of muslin

Shallow tins or dishes

METHOD

Allow the elder leaves to wilt overnight on kitchen paper to remove some of the moisture.

Tear the wilted leaves and put them along with the carrier oil into a heatproof bowl.

Place the bowl over a pan of simmering water for 3–4 hours. Keep an eye on the water level, topping up as necessary.

Once infused, the oil should turn a pale shade of green.

Strain the oil through muslin, squeezing to get every last drop. Be careful, it's hot!

Return the infused oil to the heatproof bowl over simmering water. Add the beeswax. Once melted, remove from the heat.

Allow the mixture to cool slightly, then add the essential oil and stir.

Pour into labelled shallow tins or dishes. Allow the salve to cool completely before popping on a lid.

Apply as needed.

Always do a patch test.

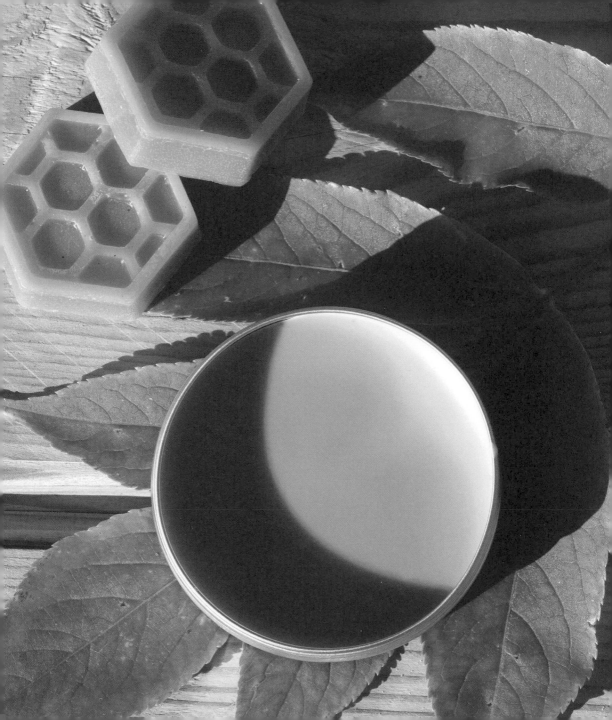

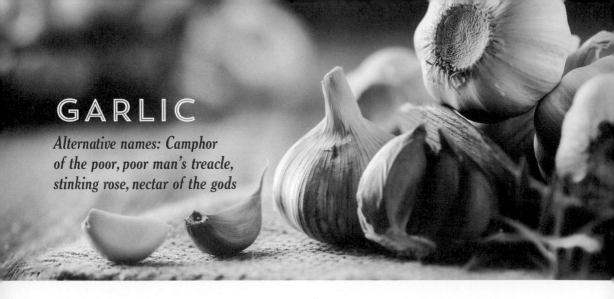

GARLIC

Alternative names: Camphor of the poor, poor man's treacle, stinking rose, nectar of the gods

HOW TO IDENTIFY: A white bulb divided into individual cloves, producing flat grass-like leaves with a very distinctive, pungent scent.

HISTORY: Garlic is believed to have originated on the shores of Mesopotamia, now known as Iraq, over 5,000 years ago. Ancient Egyptians placed it in the tombs of Pharaohs, believing that the pungent smell of garlic would protect the body from evil spirits. Workers building the pyramids were paid partly in garlic and a healthy slave was worth 6 kg of the herb. Garlic was so popular with the workers as a preferred method of payment that garlic shortages could result in all work ceasing. One year when the Nile flooded unusually high, it caused the garlic crop to fail, resulting in one of only two recorded slave revolts in ancient Egypt.

Garlic has been cultivated in Britain since the sixteenth century, when it was mostly used for medicinal purposes, the populace being very apprehensive of it as a cooking ingredient. Mrs Isabella Beeton, who famously wrote *Mrs Beeton's Book of Household Management* in 1859, did not approve of garlic as an ingredient at all, writing that garlic was *"offensive"*. That being said, she also thought that potatoes were *"suspicious"*.

During the Second World War, British agents were equipped with all sorts of clever gadgetry before they were parachuted into France. To complete their disguises, they needed to smell like true French nationals. Garlic was very unpopular among the British due to its unfamiliar taste and unfortunate effect on the breath, so Charles Fraser-Smith (the inspiration for Q in the Bond films) invented garlic impregnated chocolate bars to be eaten before the mission in the hope that this would make the herb's taste more palatable.

FOLKLORE: Midwives in ancient Greece believed that hanging garlic in the delivery room would protect mother and baby from evil spirits.

To ward off vampires, wear a garland of garlic around your neck. As an extra precaution, hang it in windows and rub it around keyholes and chimneys, too.

It was believed that garlic protected maidens from evil nymphs, warded off witches, kept away the plague and even prevented others from overtaking you or your horse in a race. Dreaming about eating garlic means that you will discover hidden secrets that may cause domestic strife. To dream that you have garlic in the house will bring you good luck.

FOLK MEDICINE: In the seventeenth century, when Nicholas Culpeper wrote his famous herbal, garlic was clearly an important medicine for many ailments, including *"any plague, sore, or foul ulcers; takes away spots and blemishes in the skin, eases pain in the ears, ripens and breaks imposthumes [abscesses] or other swellings [...] It is also held good in hydropick [water retention] diseases, the jaundice, falling sickness [epilepsy], cramps, convulsions and piles."*

Louis Pasteur, the French chemist and microbiologist, wrote of the antibacterial properties of garlic juice as early as 1858. It was then proven to be incredibly effective when used to treat an outbreak of cholera, typhoid fever and diphtheria in Beirut in 1918.

Garlic was used in the trenches of the First World War with some success. Although penicillin was in use by the Second World War, the Russian army continued to treat wounded soldiers with garlic juice, resulting in its being known as "Russian penicillin".

OTHER COMMON USES: Garlic is used to flavour many foods, vinaigrettes, sauces, marinades and, of course, garlic bread.

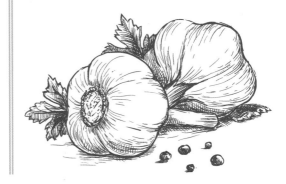

GARLIC- AND LEMON-INFUSED HONEY

Raw honey is a powerful home remedy in its own right, helping to soothe sore throats with its gentle antibacterial properties. Lemon juice is high in vitamin C, which can shorten the duration of a cold, while garlic is both antibiotic and immune boosting. This makes for quite the powerful combination.

INGREDIENTS

5 cloves of pesticide-free garlic

Juice of 1 lemon

Raw honey

Equipment needed

Small sterilized jar

METHOD

Roughly chop the garlic cloves and put them into a small clean jar. We're aiming for the jar to be about ⅔ full of garlic.

Add the lemon juice.

Pour over enough honey to fill the jar.

Shake well and allow to stand for at least three days.

Add 1 tbsp of your infused honey to hot water for a soothing drink, or take 1 tsp neat as needed.

This will keep indefinitely, although the honey may crystallize over time. If this happens, gently warm the jar up in a hot water bath until the honey melts.

Raw honey should not be consumed by children under the age of two.

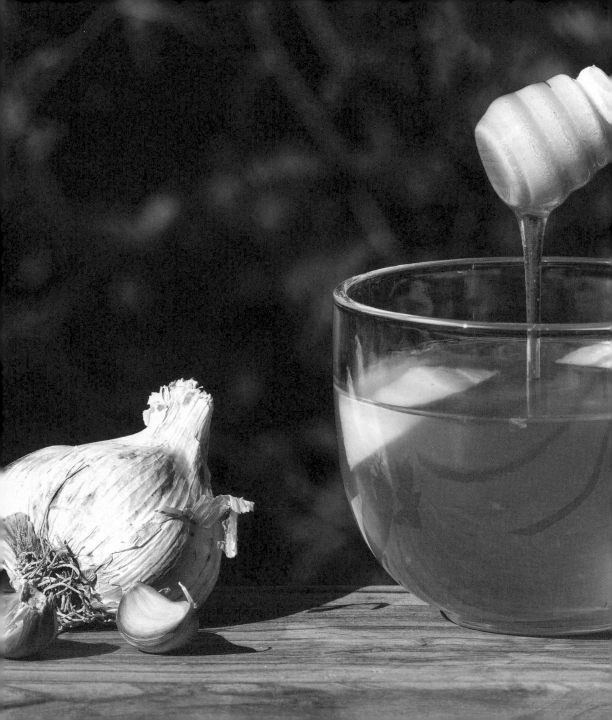

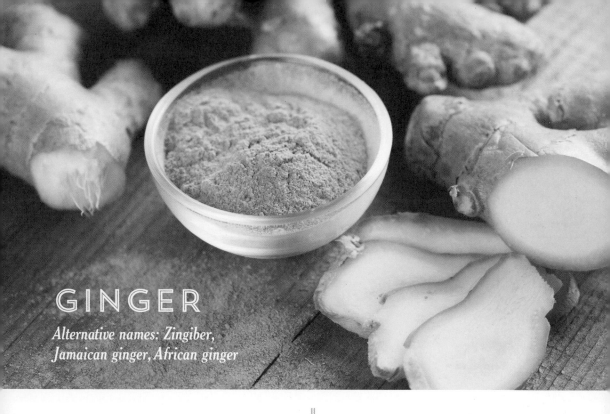

GINGER

*Alternative names: Zingiber,
Jamaican ginger, African ginger*

HOW TO IDENTIFY: A thick branched rhizome growing underground, ginger is light brown on the outside and lemon yellow on the inside. It has a sweet, spicy smell and a taste that mellows with cooking.

HISTORY: As early as 500 BCE, the Chinese philosopher Confucius was a great believer in the healing properties of ginger and reportedly ate ginger at every meal. To the Ancient Romans, ginger symbolized fertility and wealth, while the Greeks were already using the spice to make gingerbread.

As well as being used as a remedy, ginger was placed on the medieval dining table as a condiment along with salt and pepper.

By the reign of King Henry VIII in the sixteenth century, ginger was well known throughout Britain, although, as with many spices, it was expensive and only to be found on the tables of the rich. As well as enjoying many dishes that included ginger, King Henry was advised to take ginger to ward off the plague. Henry's daughter, Elizabeth I, who is credited with inventing the gingerbread man, encouraged her fleet to carry ginger plants to the new world colonies of the Caribbean where it could be grown much more economically for the British market. The Elizabethan playwright William Shakespeare was definitely a big fan: *"Had I but a penny in the world, thou shouldst have it for gingerbread."* (*Love's Labour's Lost*)

By the nineteenth century, ginger was sprinkled into beer to create ginger ale. In a practice known as "gingering", older or sick horses had ginger inserted into their rectums to make them carry their tails high and appear younger in the show ring.

FOLKLORE: Ginger has a fiery taste and was therefore believed to be a high-energy substance. As such, it was used to speed up spells and charms designed to attract love, money and success.

Islanders in Papua New Guinea are known to spit ginger into the wind in the belief that it will prevent potentially damaging storms at sea.

Chewing on ginger will give you confidence, sleeping with ginger under your bed will prevent nightmares and using it in love potions is sure to spice up your love life.

FOLK MEDICINE: On Thursday 20 July 1665, at the height of the plague in London, the diarist Samuel Pepys was given a bottle of "plague water" as a preventative measure. He writes: *"My lady Carteret did this day give me a bottle of plague water home with me."* Among ingredients such as sage, nutmeg and rue, she includes *"½ oz of ginger"*. Sadly, the recipe was unlikely to prevent infection by the plague.

Ginger tea helps to alleviate nausea and indigestion, especially during pregnancy, and the root is a powerful antiviral substance, useful to combat colds and flu.

OTHER COMMON USES: Adding fresh ginger to a footbath can treat fungal infections and bacteria on the feet as well as having a lovely warming effect.

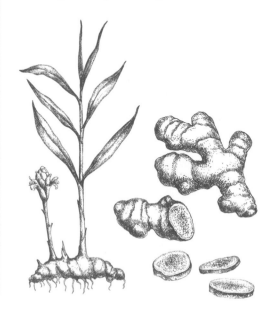

GINGER AND PINEAPPLE SMOOTHIE

If you have a sensitive stomach, bloating or just need a bit of a health boost, smoothies are easy to make as well as being delicious. The flavour of ginger marries well with pineapple, with the added bonus of being an anti-inflammatory and helping to relieve pain.

Serves two

INGREDIENTS

300 ml dairy or
plant-based milk

200 g frozen or fresh
pineapple chunks

1 banana, roughly chopped

1 tbsp ginger root, peeled
and roughly chopped

½ tsp turmeric powder
or 1 tsp fresh turmeric
root, chopped

Equipment needed

Blender

METHOD

Put all ingredients into a blender, then blitz until smooth and creamy.

Pour into two glasses.

Drink immediately.

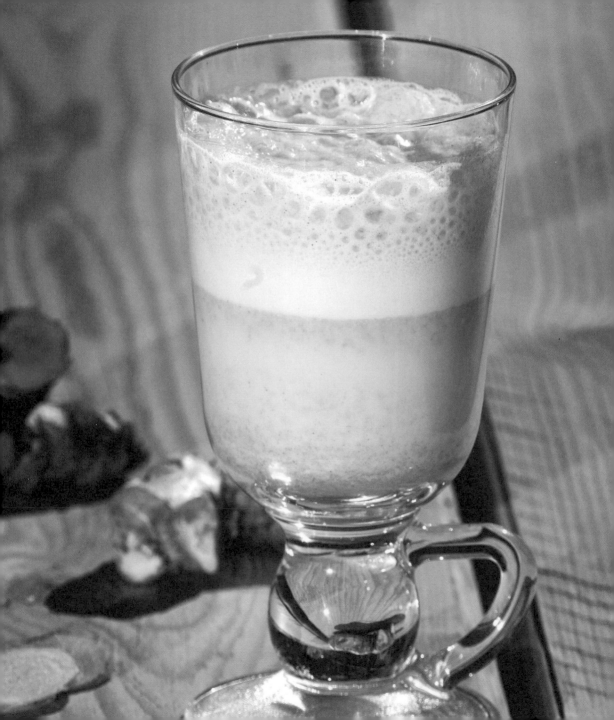

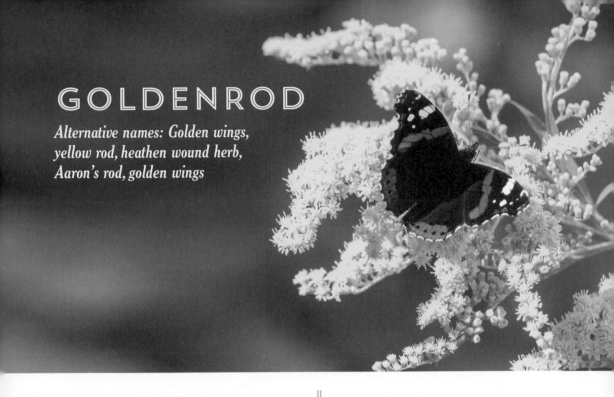

GOLDENROD

Alternative names: Golden wings, yellow rod, heathen wound herb, Aaron's rod, golden wings

HOW TO IDENTIFY: Goldenrod is a member of the daisy family with conical flower heads made up of many small bright yellow daisy-like flowers. Growing to about 1 metre (3 feet) tall, it prefers a sunny spot and will flower from late summer all the way through to early autumn.

HISTORY: Originating in the Middle East, goldenrod was imported into Europe in the sixteenth century, making it yet another herb that was incredibly expensive to buy. Botanist William Turner, who served at the court of King Henry VIII, considered goldenrod to be "*one of the best healing herbs ever discovered*". Meanwhile, his fellow herbalist John Gerard was disgusted at the price that goldenrod commanded in London: "*I have known the dry herb which came from beyond the sea sold in Bucklesbury London for half a crown an ounce.*" Shortly after, goldenrod was found growing wild in Hampstead wood and Gerard reported that since this discovery "*no man will give half a crown for a hundredweight of it*".

FOLKLORE: In New England, "rheumaty buds" containing goldenrod gall grubs (larvae laid by the goldenrod gall fly) were gathered by European settlers and popped into pockets in the belief that as long as the grub stayed alive the carrier wouldn't suffer from rheumatism.

Wear a sprig of goldenrod and you will meet your future partner the following day.

Use goldenrod when searching for hidden springs of water – the stalks will bend when water is beneath your feet.

Goldenrod flowers sprinkled in your purse or wallet will bring you riches.

FOLK MEDICINE: Known as "wound-weed" in medieval England, goldenrod was used to heal all kinds of wounds and cuts. In Scotland, goldenrod was made into an ointment to be applied to fractures.

In the seventeenth century, Culpeper wrote that goldenrod could be used to treat *"sores or ulcers in the mouth, throat, or privy parts of man or woman. The decoction also helps to fasten the teeth that are loose in the gums."*

By the twentieth century, British author Doris E. Coates recorded how *"goldenrod was always grown in the herb patch and used for wound healing, as well as a variety of other complaints. An infusion of the leaves was used for scratches, or the fresh leaf could be pressed on the injury... The infusion could also be drunk for indigestion."*

OTHER USES: In the USA in the 1920s, Thomas Edison discovered that goldenrod naturally contained rubber. He created his own cultivation and fertilization technique that maximized the rubber content in the plants, enabling goldenrod to grow to a massive 3.7 metres tall, yielding 12 per cent rubber! He even managed to put rubber tyres on the model T given to him by Henry Ford. Sadly, Edison died before he could commercially produce tyres from goldenrod and the project faded away. However, samples of one-hundred-year-old goldenrod rubber are kept in his laboratory and are still elastic and in good condition after all this time.

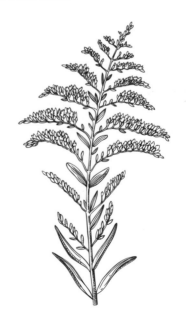

GOLDENROD WATERCOLOUR PAINT

Inks and watercolour paints can be extracted from all sorts of plant material, a great activity to do with children who can then create their own masterpiece using natural paintbrushes.

Unsurprisingly, goldenrod flowers and leaves yield a gorgeous rich golden colour, perfect for sunny day paintings.

Try red cabbage or elderberry for purple paint, beetroot for red, walnut shells for brown and leafy greens or red onion skins for green watercolour paints.

INGREDIENTS

A good handful of goldenrod leaves and flowers

Water

2 tbsp vinegar

1 tbsp salt

Equipment needed

An old pan

Muslin or tea towel

Jar

METHOD

Chop the golden rod into small pieces with scissors and place into a large pan. It is best to use an old one, just in case it gets stained.

Add enough water to cover the goldenrod completely and bring to the boil.

Add the vinegar and salt, then turn the heat down to a simmer.

After 15 minutes, check the colour by brushing some of the liquid onto white paper. Keep simmering until you reach the desired depth of colour – but be careful not to let the pan boil dry!

Allow the liquid to cool, then strain the liquid through a piece of muslin or tea towel into a clean jam jar. Compost the plant material if you can.

Keep the watercolour paint in the fridge and use within a couple of days.

To make your goldenrod paint last longer, add a few drops of essential oil of wintergreen (available in art shops) and shake.

Encourage the children to choose plants from the garden to turn into delightful natural paintbrushes. All you need is a stick, some twine and lots of imagination.

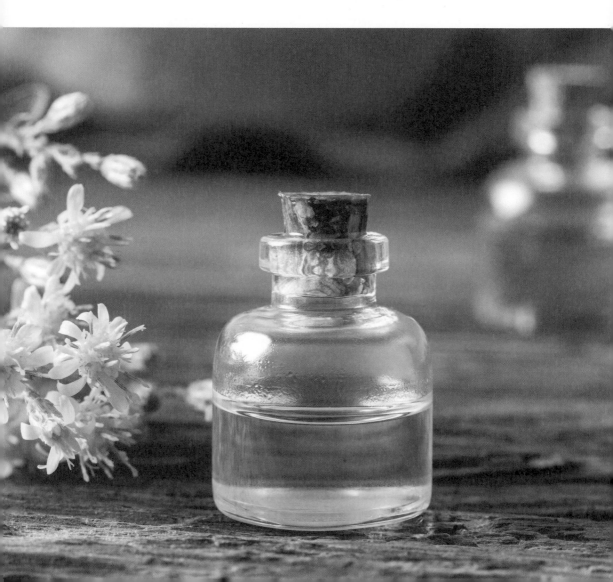

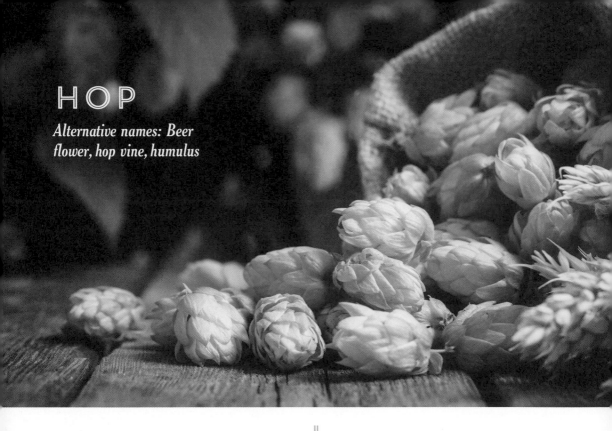

HOP

Alternative names: Beer flower, hop vine, humulus

HOW TO IDENTIFY: With its distinctive yellow-green flowers appearing between July and September, you may be lucky enough to find wild hops growing in the hedgerows. The female flowers develop into a cone-shaped fruit that turns from green to brown as it ripens, giving off a scent similar to that of garlic or yeast.

HISTORY: I was lucky enough to gather some first-hand hop-picking history from my lovely mother-in-law Janet who, as a child in the late 1940s and early 1950s, regularly went hop picking with her mother and grandmother in Kent.

Janet tells me that they slept in red tin huts on beds that they had to stuff with straw – not very comfortable at all. Although they were very poor, some families even wallpapered the walls of the huts in an effort to make them more homely. Janet has fond memories of hearing the rain pattering on the tin roof as they slept, the big kettle boiling away outside on the fire and, most of all, the wonderful community spirit that nurtured many long-lasting friendships and even love affairs; Janet's aunt Sylvia met her husband-to-be John while working in the hop fields.

Men on tall stilts walked between the hop bines pulling them down so that the women and older children could remove the hops and put them into a bushel. A "measureman" would check that the hops were cleanly picked without leaves, followed along by a "tally lady", who would mark your card with the number of bushels –very important because this was your record for payment.

Mechanized hop pickers were introduced in the 1950s, sadly putting an end to the tradition of hop picking by hand, but Janet remembers the experience as "one of the best times of my life".

FOLKLORE: If a well-dressed stranger happens to pass the hop-yard, they are seized by the pickers, tumbled into the bin, covered with leaves and not released until they have paid a fine!

Author George Orwell went hop picking in 1931. In his diary for 19 September, he recalls:

"On the last morning, when we had picked the last field, there was a queer game of catching the women and putting them in the bins… it is evidently an old custom and all harvests have some custom of this kind attached to them."

FOLK MEDICINE: In the seventeenth century, Culpeper prescribed hops for numerous ailments, including *"the French diseases [syphilis] and all manner of scabs, itch and other breakings out of the body"*.

During his reign from 1760 to 1820, King George III made use of the soporific qualities of hops by having his mattress filled with them. Hops are often included in the stuffing of modern pillows for this very reason.

Medicinally, hops were used as a poultice for arthritis and sore joints, as well as a cure for earache, toothache and boils.

OTHER COMMON USES: Hops have been used in the brewing industry since the seventeenth century. They not only give beer its distinctive flavour but also act as a preservative and to help retain its head of foam.

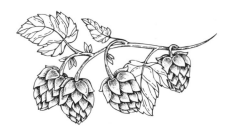

SPARKLING HOPS WATER

My recipe for sparkling hops water is alcohol free, sugar free, refreshing and something a little bit different to drink on a summer's evening. Dried hops are readily available online or in brewing shops – look for organic ones if possible.

Serves two

INGREDIENTS

500 ml filtered or bottled water

1 tbsp dried hops

Lemon juice

Sparkling water

Equipment needed

Heatproof jug

Sieve

METHOD

Boil the filtered or bottled water then allow it to cool for a couple of minutes. We're aiming for the temperature to be around 75°C (170°F).

Put the hops into a heatproof jug.

Pour over the cooled water and stir.

Leave to steep for 5–10 minutes, depending on how strong you want the flavour to be.

Strain out the hops. Compost them if you can.

Add a squeeze of lemon juice, stir the mixture and pop it into the fridge to cool completely.

For a refreshing drink, dilute 1 part hop water to 2 parts sparkling water.

Put the rest of your undiluted hop tea in a jar in the fridge where it will last for about five days.

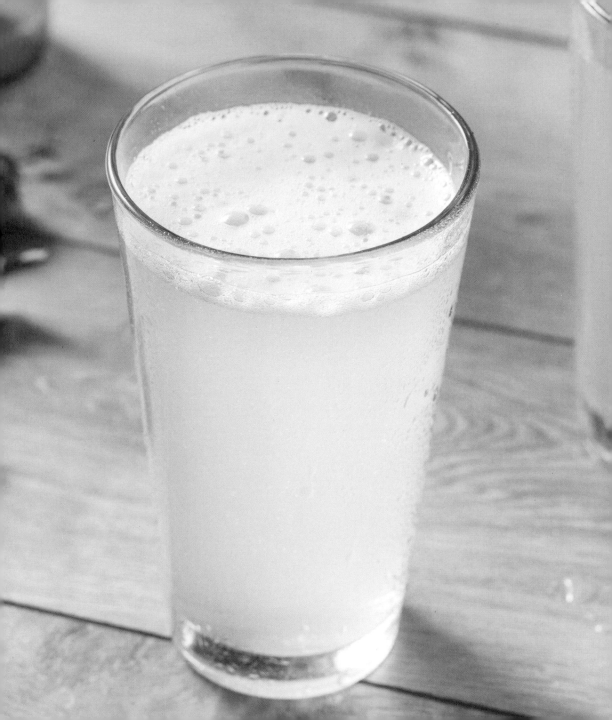

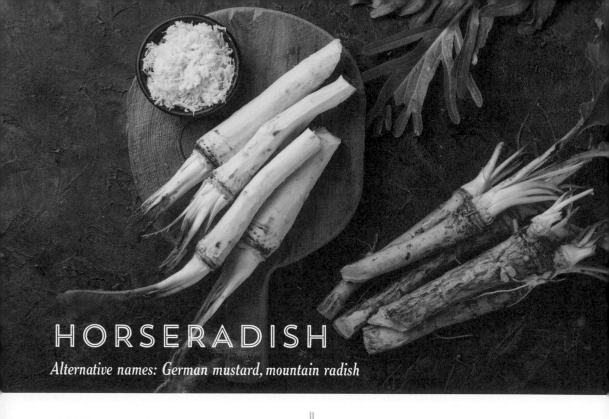

HORSERADISH

Alternative names: German mustard, mountain radish

HOW TO IDENTIFY: Mainly grown for its extremely pungent root, horseradish has large crinkled oval leaves and clusters of small white flowers.

HISTORY: The use of horseradish as both a food and a medicine by the Ancient Greeks and Egyptians dates as far back as 1500 BCE. In Greek mythology, the Oracle of Delphi tells the god Apollo that *"the radish is worth its weight in lead, the beet its weight in silver, the horseradish its weight in gold".*

Horseradish eventually made its way to central Europe via trade routes, and initially grew wild on wasteland in Britain before finding its rightful place in apothecaries and kitchens by the fifteenth century.

The English embraced the fiery heat of horseradish, and by the seventeenth century it could be found served regularly with beef and oysters. It was even incorporated into a cordial that would revive exhausted travellers – only for working men and women, though. It was far too pungent for the delicate stomachs of the upper classes.

FOLKLORE: In the Fenlands of eastern England, horseradish was used to predict the sex of an unborn child. A root was placed under the pillow of each parent, and if the root turned black under the father's pillow first, it would be a baby boy. If the root under the mother's pillow turned black first, then it would be a girl.

Angry or depressed people were advised to wrap horseradish leaves around their feet. This was believed to draw the angry heat away from the head and make them calm again.

Horseradish root combined with lemon juice applied to the skin was recommended to remove freckles. Alternatively, slice some root into milk and then splash on your face to improve the complexion.

FOLK MEDICINE: Medieval folk used the leaves and roots of horseradish to treat a variety of ailments including sore throats, coughs, asthma, toothache, chilblains and digestive upsets.

Horseradish was rubbed onto bald heads to stimulate hair growth and applied as a poultice to ease sciatica, headaches and gout.

Herbalist John Gerard claimed that horse-radish *"relieved colic, increased urination, and killed worms in children".*

Seventeenth-century herbalist William Coles highly recommended that horseradish be carried aboard ships on long voyages as a remedy for scurvy, a condition caused by lack of vitamin C.

On Friday 16 September 1664, Samuel Pepys recalled how he drank *"a cup of horse-radish ale"* on the recommendation of an acquaintance whose friend had been *"troubled with the stone".*

British botanists Robert Bentley and Henry Trimen wrote in their 1880 book, *Medicinal Plants,* how *"grated horseradish root was mixed with honey and warm water for influenza, and it could be used as a poultice by adding corn starch to fresh horseradish and applying it to the affected areas in a gauze bandage".*

Horseradish leaves can be rubbed on nettle stings in the same way that you would use dock or plantain.

OTHER COMMON USES: Horseradish sauce has long been a favoured condiment to accompany roast beef for a traditional Sunday dinner.

I was also fascinated to read that a smoke detector has been developed for the hearing-impaired which sprays pungent horseradish into the air, waking even the deepest of sleepers.

HORSERADISH AND APPLE SINUS REMEDY

If you have ever eaten horseradish, then you'll know how quickly it affects your sinuses, setting your eyes watering and your nose running relentlessly. That's exactly the effect that we want to harness for this head-clearing remedy.

This recipe is not one for the faint-hearted, small children, pregnant or hot-flushing ladies, but it will clear nasal congestion effectively.

INGREDIENTS

A thumb-sized piece of fresh horseradish root

1 organic sweet eating apple

3 tbsp raw honey

3 tbsp raw apple cider vinegar

1 tsp fine sea salt

Equipment needed

Blender

Sterilized jar

METHOD

Peel and grate the horseradish.

Grate the apple (no need to peel).

Combine the two together thoroughly in a food blender.

Add honey, vinegar and salt, and blend again.

Store in the fridge in a clean jar topped with a non-metallic lid.

Take a small spoonful (go carefully to start) up to three times a day to clear sinuses and ease congestion. You can spread this remedy on crackers with cheese to make it more palatable if you wish.

Keeps in the fridge for up to three months.

The Herbal Apothecary

Horseradish &
Apple Remedy

LAVENDER

Alternative names: Nard, spike, elf leaf, spikenard

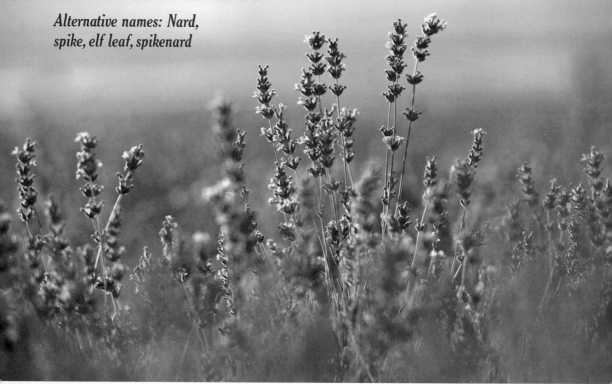

HOW TO IDENTIFY: Delicate purple flowers, with a characteristic camphor-like scent, sit on top of long thin stems.

HISTORY: Still-fragrant lavender was found in the tomb of Tutankhamun, and it is believed that Cleopatra used the heady scent of lavender to help her seduce the Roman politician and general Mark Antony.

Used in bath houses during Roman times, "lavender" comes from the Latin word *"lavare"*, meaning "to wash". Lavender gave the bathwater a lovely perfume and helped to restore the natural glow of the skin. The Romans introduced lavender to Britain to ward off the lice and fleas that they discovered were prolific among the native population.

FOLKLORE: Drinking lavender tea at bedtime on St Luke's Day (18 October) while reciting the charm *"St Luke, St Luke, be kind to me, in my dreams, let me my true love see"* will reveal a future husband.

Adding lavender to the bathwater of bewitched children will drive out their demons. Hanging lavender above your doorway or burning an incense of lavender, frankincense, basil, rue and lemon balm will protect your home from further unwanted visitors.

In the nineteenth century, ladies wore small lavender pouches in their cleavage to attract suitors.

FOLK MEDICINE: Culpeper recommended that lavender, a herb of many uses, be combined with *"hore hound, fennel and asparagus root, and a little cinnamon [...] to help the falling sickness [epilepsy] and the giddiness or turning of the brain: to gargle the mouth with the decoction thereof is good against the toothache".*

Lavender oil was massaged into paralyzed limbs to stimulate movement, while oleumspicoe, made by mixing lavender oil with turpentine, was massaged into stiff joints and sprains.

OTHER COMMON USES: Lavender is a well-known aid to restful sleep and can be found in many skin care products for its anti-inflammatory and antibacterial properties that calm and heal acne and eczema.

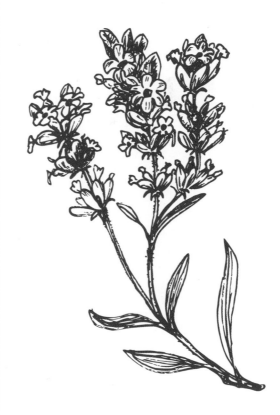

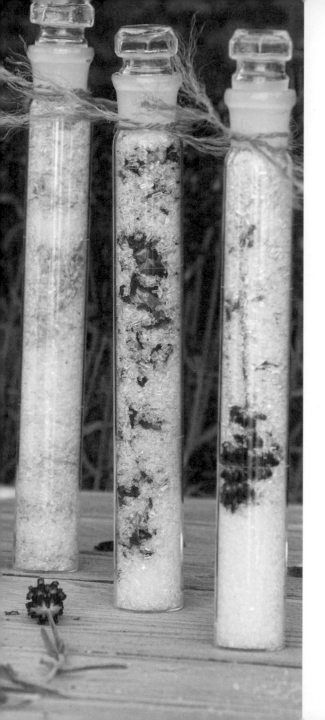

LAVENDER BATH SHOTS

Nothing is better for the body and the soul than to have a long hot bath at the end of a stressful day. Epsom salts contain magnesium and sulphates that are absorbed through the skin, believed to help in the removal of toxins, to relax tired muscles and soften the skin. Himalayan pink salt, believed to be the purest salt on earth, helps balance the pH of the skin. The scent of lavender helps to lift your mood, calms the mind and just helps you to unwind.

I was lucky enough to find these beautiful glass test tubes in a local charity shop, but you can easily find them online. The bath shots look just as pretty in upcycled glass jars, too.

INGREDIENTS

125 g Epsom salts

60 g Himalayan pink
salt, finely ground

10 drops lavender
essential oil

Handful of dried lavender

Equipment needed

Sterilized glass test
tubes or jars

METHOD

Combine the Epsom salts, pink salt and lavender oil in a bowl. You can mix them as much or as little as you like.

Stir in the lavender flowers – they also look lovely layered with the salts.

Pop the mixture into test tubes or glass jars and seal tightly.

Add the shots to running bathwater, stirring to dissolve.

Relax.

Try using dried calendula, rose or camomile flowers, changing your essential oil to match.

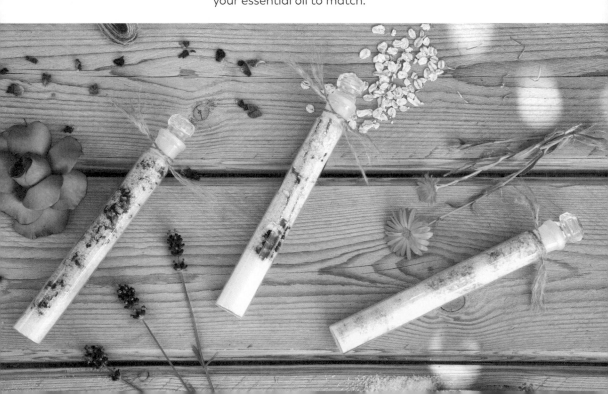

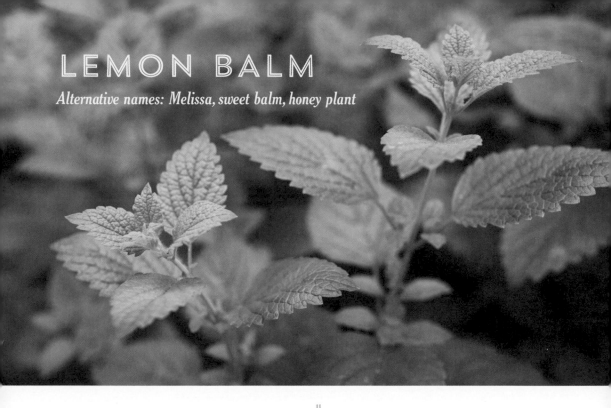

LEMON BALM

Alternative names: Melissa, sweet balm, honey plant

HOW TO IDENTIFY: Lemon balm is a characteristically square-stemmed member of the mint family. Run your hands through this herb and you'll release the sharp lemony scent that gives this herb its name. Growing up to 80 cm (31 in.) it is tall and bushy. Lemon balm is such a resilient perennial herb that once you have a plant in your garden, you can enjoy it for life.

HISTORY: Lemon balm was planted near beehives in ancient Turkey and around the Greek temple of Artemis to keep the sacred honeybees happy and discourage them from swarming. The citrusy herb was brought to Europe via the Spanish trade routes, where it made its way into monastery gardens to be used medicinally.

The Knights Templar tied a sprig of lemon balm onto the handle of their swords in the belief that it would heal any wounds that they suffered during battle.

According to The London Dispensary, a clinic founded in 1696 to give medicines to those who couldn't afford them, lemon balm would *"renew youth, strengthen the brain and reduce baldness"* as well as being able to *"revivify a man".*

FOLKLORE: Carry a sprig of lemon balm around with you to attract love. If that fails, a potent love potion can be made by soaking the herb in wine and sharing it with your prospective partner.

FOLK MEDICINE: In the medieval period, lemon balm was used as a treatment for a rabid dog bite, for boils and spots, as a cure for baldness and for easing the pain of toothache.

Monks and nuns famously used lemon balm to make Carmelite water, which consists of wine infused with herbs, as a cure for headaches, digestive complaints and to lift the spirits.

In the seventeenth century, Culpeper recommended the use of lemon balm for *"weak stomachs, to cause the heart to become merry, to help digestion, to open obstructions to the brain, and to expel melancholy vapours from the heart and arteries".*

In the twentieth century, herbalist Maud Grieve explained how lemon balm steeped in wine *"comforts the heart and drives away melancholy and sadness".*

OTHER COMMON USES: An infusion of lemon balm can be sprayed onto plants to repel insects, and keeping a bunch of lemon balm on your windowsill discourages flies and insects from entering your home.

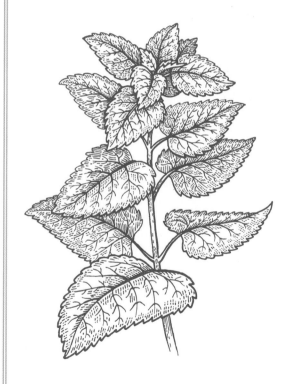

LEMON BALM FOR LIPS

Lemon balm has powerful antiviral properties which are useful when applied topically to prevent and banish cold sores. Cold sores usually appear when we become tired or stressed. Try to boost your immune system and look after yourself so that hopefully cold sores won't be an ongoing problem.

Pick your lemon balm as fresh as possible. It should be bright green and free from any brown spots.

Makes approx. 50 ml

INGREDIENTS

2 tbsp lemon-balm-infused carrier oil (see page 14)

1 tbsp natural beeswax or soy pellets

1 tbsp organic coconut oil

10 drops tea tree essential oil

Equipment needed

Small tins or shallow dishes

METHOD

Gently melt the lemon-balm-infused oil, beeswax and coconut oil in a heatproof bowl, placed over a pan of boiling water.

Once melted, take the mixture off the heat and stir in the essential oil.

Pour into small tins or shallow dishes and allow to cool completely before putting on the lids.

Should last nine months.

Substitute 10 drops of lemon balm essential oil in 2 tbsp carrier oil for lemon-balm-infused oil if you need a quick remedy for cold sores.

Lemon balm is not recommended if you are taking sedatives or thyroid medication.

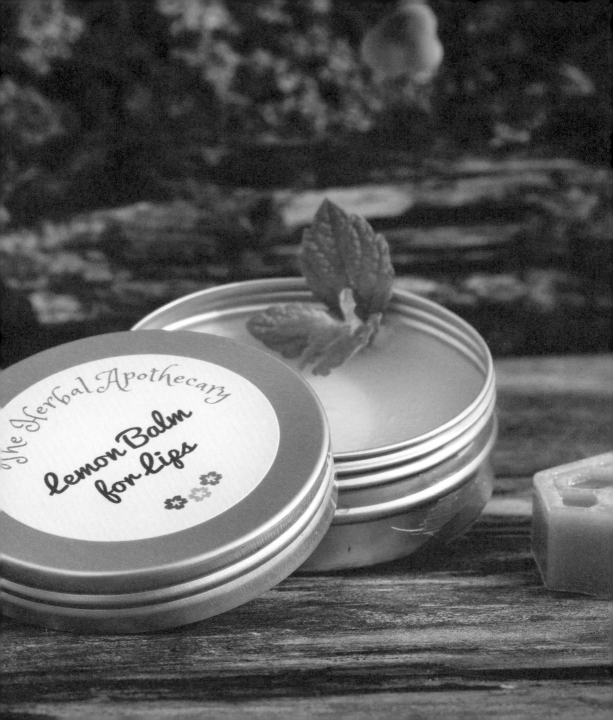

The Herbal Apothecary

lemon Balm
for lips

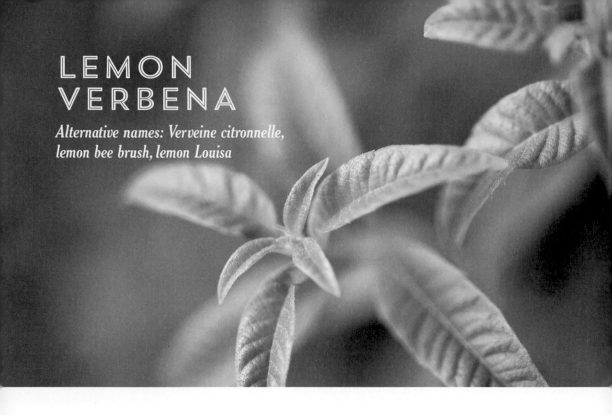

LEMON VERBENA

Alternative names: Verveine citronnelle, lemon bee brush, lemon Louisa

HOW TO IDENTIFY: The pale green spear-like leaves of lemon verbena smell incredibly citrusy when crushed, reminiscent of the sherbet lemon sweets of my childhood.

HISTORY: Lemon verbena wasn't known in Britain until the eighteenth century, when it was imported by the Spanish specifically for use in the perfumery industry. By the end of the nineteenth century, this herb could be found all over Europe in greenhouses and indoor gardens, ready to be used as a flavouring substitute for lemons and distilled into oil for the cosmetics industry.

Victorian ladies placed the leaves in their handkerchiefs and inhaled the scent to revive them when overcome by the tightness of their corsets.

FOLKLORE: Ancient Greeks slept with lemon verbena under their pillows to give them sweet dreams or drank lemon verbena tea to make them "as strong as Titan".

116

Wearing a sprig of lemon verbena will make you more attractive to a potential partner, most probably because you will smell delicious!

The cleansing properties of lemon verbena have historically been used to purify altars, while bathing with lemon verbena leaves will rid you of any evil influences.

Lemon verbena is notoriously difficult to propagate from cuttings and it was believed that "anyone who can make cuttings of lemon verbena grow will not die unmarried".

FOLK MEDICINE: The Incas are believed to have been the first people to discover the wonderful medicinal benefits of lemon verbena. They used it to help balance gut bacteria and reduce flatulence as well as harnessing its antioxidant, anti-inflammatory and anti-anxiety properties.

Since lemon verbena didn't reach European shores until the eighteenth century, it wasn't known to the seventeenth-century herbalist Culpeper, so unfortunately little historical medicinal use from that period is recorded.

Lemon verbena tea helps with digestion, trapped wind, insomnia and gout, and can be drunk to relieve colds and fevers. The scent of lemon verbena can be uplifting, calm the nerves and help to release muscle tension.

OTHER COMMON USES: This herb is used for its incredible scent by the famous French cosmetic producer L'Occitane in their lemon verbena range of shower gels, eau de toilette and many other products.

The leaves of lemon verbena can be placed among linens to keep them smelling fresh and repel insects, moths and flies.

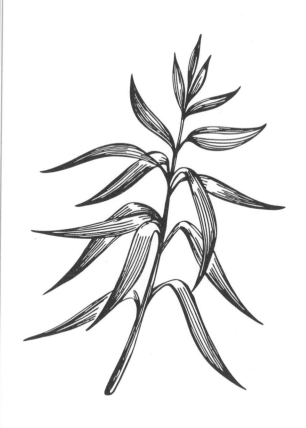

LEMON VERBENA SUGAR

I simply adore the flavour of fresh lemon verbena and wanted to create something that would preserve its essence so that I could use it all year round. Lemon verbena sugar does just this and can be sprinkled on fresh fruit or made into a delicious zingy cake that everyone will love.

INGREDIENTS

225 g fair-trade
caster sugar

25 g young tender lemon
verbena leaves – older
leaves can be stringy

Equipment needed

Stick blender or small
food processor

Pestle and mortar
or rolling pin

METHOD

Remove the leaves from their stalks.

Put the sugar into a bowl and add the verbena leaves.

Blitz either using a stick blender or a small food processor until all the leaves are chopped finely and your sugar has turned an attractive shade of green.

Spread the sugar onto a sheet of baking paper and put it somewhere warm for 24 hours or until it is completely dry.

Break up any clumps with a pestle and mortar or the end of a rolling pin.

Pour the sugar into an airtight container. Use within six months.

TO MAKE LEMON VERBENA ICING SUGAR:

Using a stick blender, blitz 10–15 g of tender lemon verbena leaves with 225 g sifted icing sugar in a large bowl. Add the juice of a lemon gradually until you get a thick spreading consistency. To use: pour into the middle of the cake, spreading it across the surface with a wet palette knife to cover.

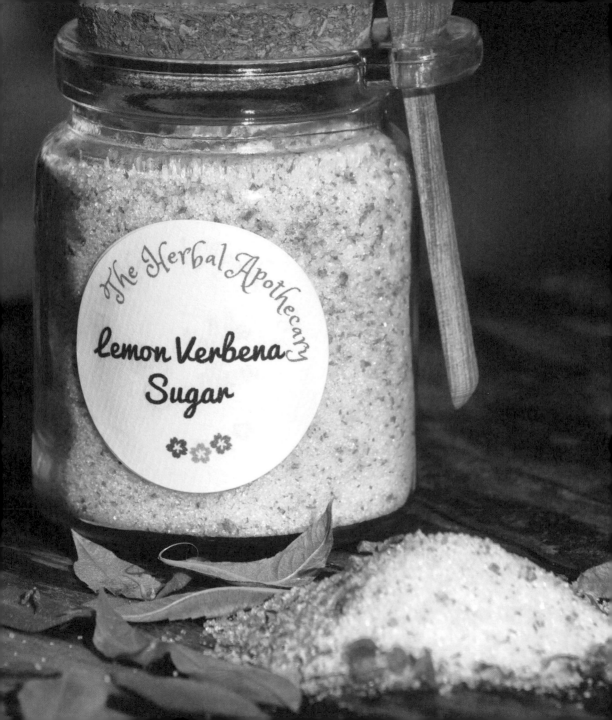

The Herbal Apothecary

Lemon Verbena
Sugar

✿ ✿ ✿

LEMON VERBENA TRAY BAKE

Serves 10–12 people

INGREDIENTS

225 g lemon verbena sugar

225 g self-raising flour

225 g softened butter

1 level tsp baking powder

4 medium free-range eggs

Juice of 1 lemon

Zest of 2 unwaxed lemons

Equipment needed

Food mixer

30 x 23-cm cake tin

METHOD

Preheat oven to 180°C (350°F).

Grease and line a 30 x 23-cm cake tin.

Put all the ingredients into a food mixer and beat until well combined. Add a drop of milk or a plant-based alternative if the mixture seems a little stiff.

Turn the mixture out into the prepared tin and level the surface.

Bake for 35–40 minutes until the cake feels springy and has shrunk away from the sides of the tin.

Leave to cool completely.

Ice with Lemon Verbena Icing (see page 118).

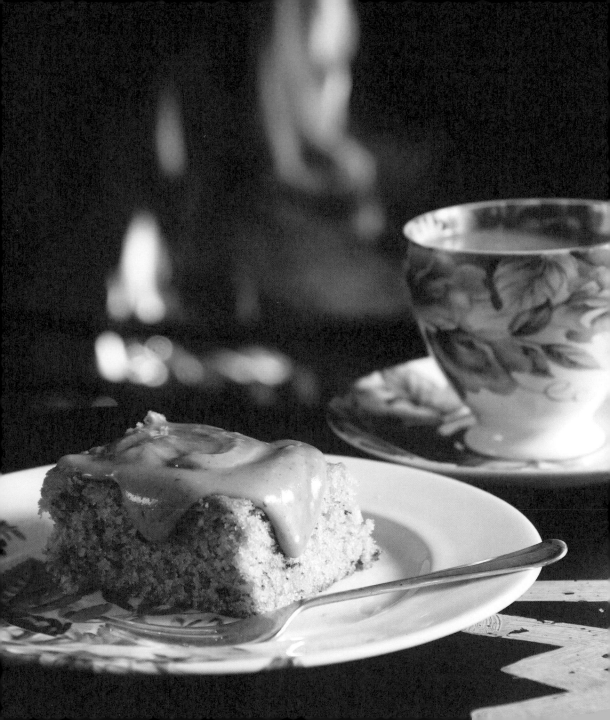

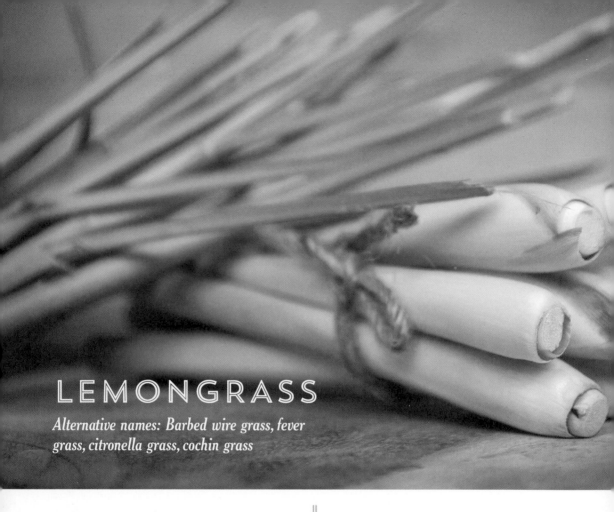

LEMONGRASS

Alternative names: Barbed wire grass, fever grass, citronella grass, cochin grass

HOW TO IDENTIFY: Lemongrass is a perennial herb that grows in stiff clumps of upright stems similar to spring onions – but with a beautiful fresh citrusy scent.

HISTORY: Lemongrass has been cultivated in southern India and Sri Lanka for at least 5,000 years, where it was used for medicinal and culinary purposes and also as a fragrance to disguise body odour.

Lemongrass essential oil was unknown outside of Asia until the seventeenth century, when it was exported to Europe for use in the perfume industry. Only the very rich could afford lemongrass oil and it became the scent of the upper class.

In the twenty-first century, lemongrass is one of the most used essential oils and is available worldwide.

FOLKLORE: Planting lemongrass around the boundaries of your property will keep serpents, evil spirits and dragons away.

Take a bath with some lemongrass leaves and you will attract a lover. It will also encourage honesty, fidelity, growth and purification.

Lemongrass tea is said to improve psychic powers and give you the ability to see into the future.

Essential oil of lemongrass was also used to promote clear thinking and support memory. Its action was thought to be spiritually cleansing and as such it was used to combat jinxes and remove negative energy.

FOLK MEDICINE: In Brazil, lemongrass was traditionally used by the indigenous Kraho people for its anti-convulsant properties and to help reduce anxiety.

In East India and Sri Lanka, lemongrass was combined with other herbs to make a drink locally known as fever tea. This beverage was used to treat fevers, irregular menstruation, diarrhoea and stomach-aches.

Lemongrass is also used in India to treat fungal infections such as athlete's foot.

OTHER COMMON USES: Citronella oil, a natural insect repellent, is produced from a variety of lemongrass and is commonly used in outdoor candles.

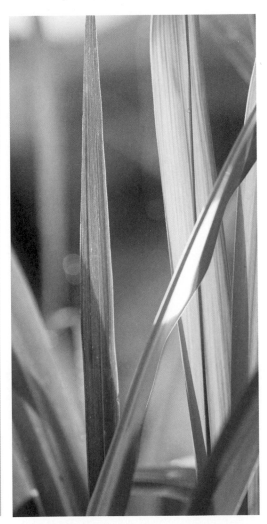

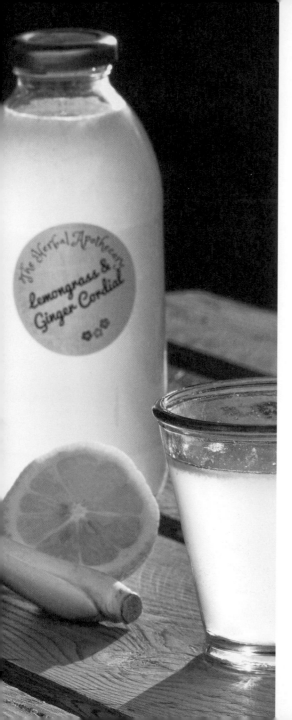

LEMONGRASS AND GINGER CORDIAL

Many of us are trying to reduce our sugar consumption. Unfortunately, shop-bought cordial is very sugar laden, as well as containing preservatives and colourings. The beauty about making your own cordials is that you have complete control over the quality and quantity of the ingredients you use. A friend gave us the most incredible lemongrass, so we combined it with fresh ginger for this refreshing, tummy-calming cordial.

Serves four

INGREDIENTS

1 litre filtered water

250 g white sugar (you can use light brown, but the resulting colour will be muddy)

6 fat lemongrass stalks, roughly chopped

300 g fresh ginger, peeled and roughly chopped

Juice of 3 lemons

Equipment needed

Stick blender

Sterilized bottle

METHOD

Place the water and sugar in a saucepan and gently heat to dissolve the sugar.

Add the lemongrass, ginger and lemon juice. Boil for 5–10 minutes until the liquid becomes syrupy.

Remove from heat and allow the flavours to infuse until the liquid is room temperature.

Using a stick blender, blitz the cordial to release maximum flavour into the liquid.

Add more sugar to taste if needed.

Strain into a clean bottle, label and chill.

Serve over ice with sparkling water and a slice of lemon.

Will last for approximately six months in a refrigerator, and longer if more sugar is added.

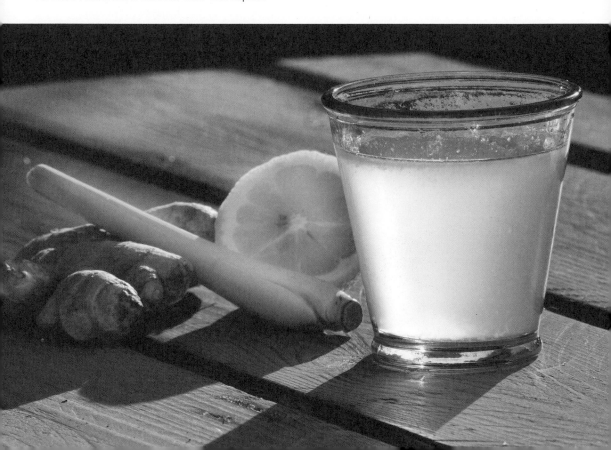

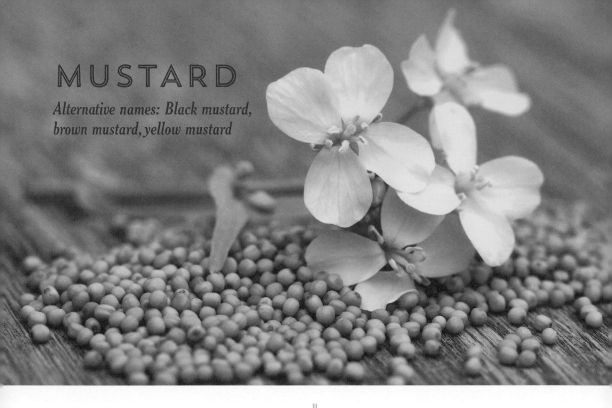

MUSTARD

Alternative names: Black mustard, brown mustard, yellow mustard

HOW TO IDENTIFY: Mustard is an annual herb grown specifically for its seeds for use in condiments. The seeds are also made into mustard oil or used as animal fodder. These seeds can be black, yellow or brown, and can be ground with liquid to create a condiment. The flowers of the plant are yellow with four petals and the leaves and stems are edible, too.

HISTORY: Black mustard originated in the Mediterranean, brown mustard from China and yellow mustard from southern Europe. The Greeks and Romans used mustard as both a medicine and a spice.

By the ninth century, European monks were making quite a profit growing and selling mustard. The first instance of mustard as a recognisable condiment occurred in the small French city of Dijon, instigated by the mustard-loving Pope John XXII of Avignon, who supposedly created the role of "Grand mustard maker to the Pope" just for his lazy nephew.

In the twelfth century, mustard seeds were ground at the table using a pestle and mortar, where their strong flavour was used to help disguise the taste of rotting meat caused by lack of refrigeration. By the fifteenth century, monks on the Farne Islands in north-east England ground the seeds using quern stones to make "*mwstert*".

Fast forward to the eighteenth century, where Mrs Clements from Durham in the north-east of England invented a revolutionary secret process using techniques borrowed from flour mills for extracting the most flavour from mustard seeds, therefore inventing English mustard. King George I was very fond of her spicy product and gave Mrs Clements many orders for her mustard. Her business then became both successful and lucrative, with people desperate to follow royal fashion.

FOLKLORE: European folklore tells us that a German bride should sew mustard seeds into the hem of her wedding dress if she wishes to be the dominant partner.

In Eastern Europe, the coffins and graves of suspected vampires were sprinkled with copious amounts of mustard seeds. According to folklore, vampires are obsessed with counting things. As such, a vampire would have to count all the seeds before they would be able to leave their grave and would either starve from lack of nourishment or be caught by the sun's deadly rays!

Sprinkle mustard seeds around the boundaries of your home to prevent demons entering your property – more counting!

FOLK MEDICINE: Sixteenth-century herbalist John Gerard recommended that *"the seed of mustard pound with vinegar, is an excellent sauce, good to be eaten with any grosse meates either fish or flesh, because it doth help digestion, warmeth the stomacke and provoketh appetite".*

His contemporary Nicholas Culpeper believed in mustard's digestive merits, too: *"let such whose stomachs are too weak they cannot digest their meat [...] take one of about half a dram of weight an hour or two before meals".*

The warming properties of mustard have long been harnessed to make poultices for chest infections, painful joints, sore muscles, bronchitis, abscesses and ulcers.

OTHER COMMON USES: Research is currently underway to find out if mustard seed oil can be used as a sustainable replacement for petrol and diesel.

WARMING MUSTARD FOOT BATH

Mustard baths were a traditional folk remedy in England for many hundreds of years. At the first sign of a cold, out would come the mustard. The natural warmth of mustard helps to sweat out a cold, Epsom salts soothe those aching muscles and bicarbonate of soda has both natural antiseptic and antifungal properties.

Combine all of this with some of your favourite essential oils and you're in for a real treat.

Makes enough for one relaxing footbath

INGREDIENTS

1 tbsp mustard powder

1 tbsp bicarbonate of soda

1½ tbsp Epsom salts

10 drops of your favourite essential oils – I like to use lavender to aid relaxation

Not recommended for small children, during pregnancy or if you are allergic to mustard.

METHOD

Mix together all the dry ingredients, making sure to break up any lumps with a fork.

Pour comfortably hot water into a large bowl. A washing-up bowl works well.

Get yourself comfy, wrap up warm, make a cup of your favourite tea and have a towel close by.

Pour the mustard mixture into the bowl, add the essential oils if you are using them and stir into the water. The bicarbonate of soda will make the water fizz.

Once you are happy that the water is not too hot, pop your bare feet in the bath and relax for 20–30 minutes, topping up with hot water as the bath cools down.

If at any time your skin begins to tingle or burn, remove your feet and rinse thoroughly with clean water.

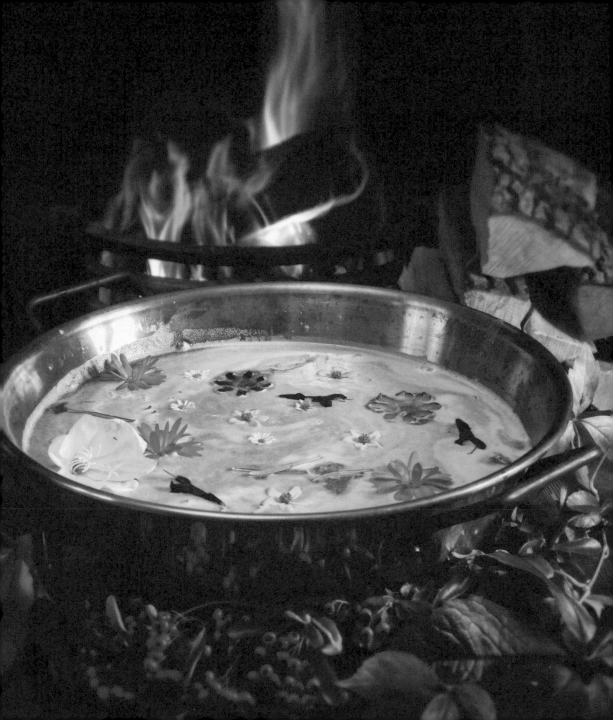

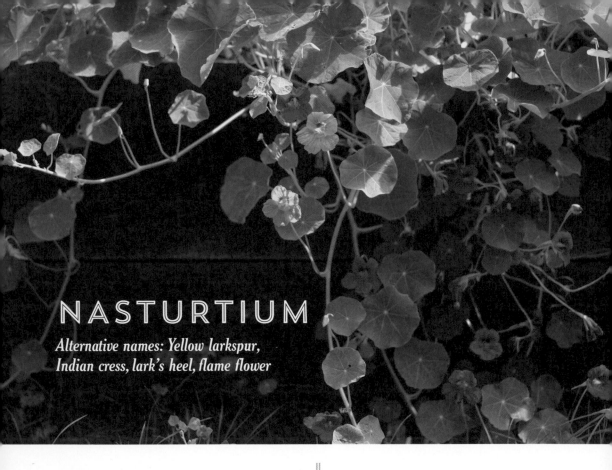

NASTURTIUM

Alternative names: Yellow larkspur,
Indian cress, lark's heel, flame flower

HOW TO IDENTIFY: Nasturtium's circular leaves are connected to a long central trailing stem. The flowers are round and blousy, coming in bright yellow, orange or dark pink. Both flowers and leaves are edible and have a distinctive peppery flavour similar to rocket.

HISTORY: Nasturtiums originate from Peru, where Jesuit missionaries noticed that the indigenous Inca people used the plant as a salad vegetable and a medicinal herb.

In the late fifteenth century, Spanish conquistadors brought nasturtium seeds to Europe for herbalists, who quickly shared the seeds with each other and spread the plant throughout Europe. Nasturtiums became especially popular after King Louis XIV planted them in the gardens of the palace of Versailles. The herb was easy to grow and provided a source of both food and spice at a time when food was scarce in France.

Thomas Jefferson, the third president of the United States, apparently loved growing nasturtiums and particularly enjoyed eating pickled nasturtium seeds.

Containing more vitamin C than many other plants, pickled nasturtium seeds were taken on board Victorian ships to prevent scurvy.

Dried and ground nasturtium seeds were used as a substitute for black pepper during the embargo of the Second World War.

FOLKLORE: The Victorians liked to use floriography, or the language of flowers, to communicate their feelings by using specific arrangements to convey coded messages to the recipient. Nasturtiums were used to represent "patriotism" and "conquest".

In fact, there seems to have always been strong links with war and conquest, perhaps because nasturtium leaves resemble the shape of a shield. In the 1800s, soldiers customarily wore nasturtium flowers given to them by maidens as a sign that they had been victorious in battle.

Plant three red nasturtiums in your garden to keep unwanted visitors away.

FOLK MEDICINE: Nasturtium leaves ground with water and then strained create a natural disinfectant wash for minor cuts and scrapes, while chewing the leaves cleanses the mouth.

The plant is high in sulphur and has natural antibiotic properties. For this reason, a tea made from the leaves can be used as a steam to help clear acne or as a final rinse to relieve dandruff.

With lots of immune-boosting vitamin C, nasturtium tea made with the leaves and flowers can ease coughs and sore throats and speed up recovery time.

OTHER COMMON USES: Nasturtiums are widely used by organic vegetable gardeners as an effective companion plant. They attract bees and other pollinators and draw potential pests like aphids away from the main crop.

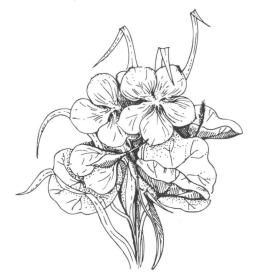

NASTURTIUM VINEGAR

This vinegar is easy to make and harnesses the lovely peppery flavours of nasturtium flowers as well as their beautiful colour. Nasturtium leaves can be used in this vinegar, too, but bear in mind that the result won't be as vibrantly coloured.

INGREDIENTS

Enough pesticide-free nasturtium flowers to loosely fill a jar

White wine vinegar or apple cider vinegar

Equipment needed

Sterilized jar

METHOD

Fill your jar with clean nasturtium flowers and cover them completely with vinegar.

Seal the jar with a non-metallic lid.

Leave the jar in a cool place for one to three weeks.

Strain out the nasturtium flowers and bottle the vinegar.

Use your peppery vinegar in salad dressings or marinades.

Lasts indefinitely.

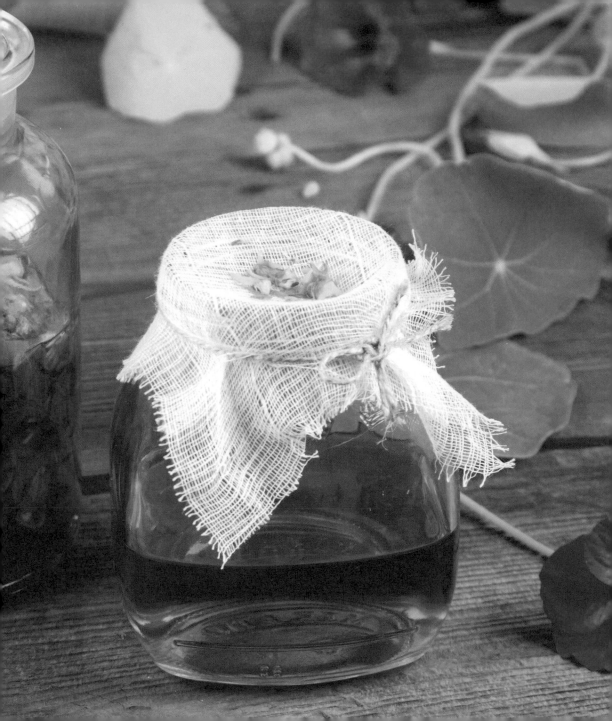

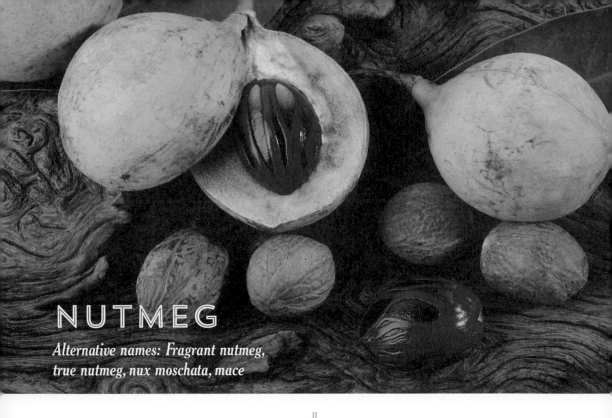

NUTMEG

Alternative names: Fragrant nutmeg, true nutmeg, nux moschata, mace

HOW TO IDENTIFY: Nutmeg is the seed found inside the ripe fruit of the nutmeg tree; the red lacy membrane that surrounds the seed is mace. Both elements have a similar warm and spicy flavour and as such can be substituted for each other in baking.

HISTORY: The nutmeg tree grows in Indonesia, Malaysia and southern India, and at one time it was the most expensive spice in the world. In the 1600s, the Dutch and the British were waging a bloody war for control of the incredibly lucrative spice trade. In 1667, the two countries finally agreed a treaty to end the bloodshed. The Dutch traded the North American island of Manhattan in exchange for the nutmeg-producing island of Run in Indonesia, as well as sugar-producing land in South America.

So why was nutmeg such a valuable commodity? It was very rare, it was rumoured to have the ability to ward off the plague and it was apparently being misused by the wealthy as a hallucinogenic.

Whole nutmeg seeds were carried by rich Europeans, who would use tiny graters to publicly grate their own nutmeg in restaurants and at each other's dinner parties as a flamboyant show of wealth.

FOLKLORE: Carry nutmeg wrapped in purple cloth in your pocket to ensure a favourable outcome in legal matters and court cases.

Sprinkling nutmeg into a woman's shoe at midnight will make her fall madly in love with you and giving her a drink flavoured with nutmeg is believed to have the same effect.

Nutmeg seems to have strong associations with love spells. You are more likely to attract a potential partner if you carry a nutmeg under your arm. To keep your partner faithful, you should first split a nutmeg fruit into four equal parts. One piece should be burned, one should be thrown off a cliff, the third piece should be buried and finally the fourth piece should be boiled in water to make a drink. Carry this last piece of nutmeg everywhere with you, even placing it under your pillow at night. Your partner will never stray.

Dreaming of nutmeg means that you will achieve great status, have a warm and loving home and that positive changes will happen in your life.

FOLK MEDICINE: A pinch of nutmeg added to warm milk at bedtime will help you sleep and aid digestion.

Combined with the herb eyebright, Culpeper wrote that *"a little mace and fennel seed and drank or eaten in a broth; or the said powder made into an electuary with sugar, and taken, has the same powerful effect to help and restore the sight decayed through age".*

OTHER COMMON USES: Nutmeg is anti-microbial and anti-inflammatory, making it the perfect remedy for acne. Simply make a paste from nutmeg and honey, apply it to your skin and leave for 20 minutes before rinsing off with warm water.

Always do a patch test.

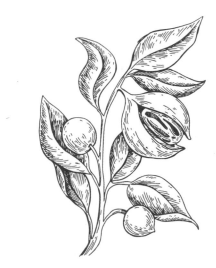

AUTUMN SPICE BLEND

As summer slowly turns into autumn, I experience a longing for certain spices, not just for their taste but for their smell, too. Nutmeg, cinnamon, cloves, allspice and ginger are evocative of cosy dark evenings in front of a log fire with a mug of hot chocolate to warm the hands and a plate of autumn spiced shortbread to warm the heart.

It's worth making up a large batch of autumn spice blend for use in cakes, biscuits and to sprinkle on hot chocolate as the nights grow longer.

INGREDIENTS

1 tsp ground nutmeg

½ tsp allspice

½ tsp ground cloves

3 tsp ground ginger

4 tsp ground cinnamon

METHOD

Add all the spices into a bowl, mix well and decant into a small, clean labelled jar.

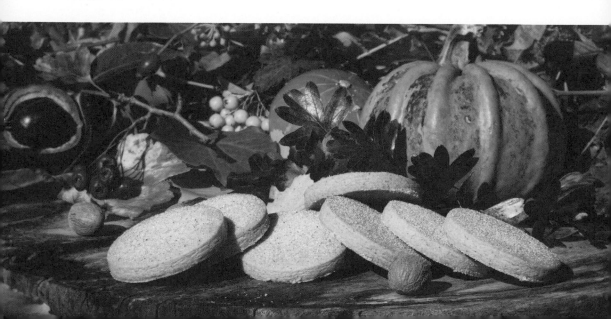

AUTUMN SPICE SHORTBREAD

Makes 20–24 delicious shortbread biscuits

INGREDIENTS

225 g softened unsalted butter or plant-based alternative

110 g golden caster sugar

225 g plain flour

110 g cornflour

3 tsp autumn spice blend

Pinch of fine sea salt

Equipment needed

2 baking trays

Cookie cutters

METHOD

Line two baking trays with baking paper and preheat oven to 170°C (340°F).

Use a mixer or wooden spoon to cream the butter and sugar until light and fluffy.

Sift in the flour, cornflour and autumn spice and add the salt.

Mix until the dough begins to clump together.

Tip out onto a floured board and gently knead to a smooth dough.

Place the dough between two sheets of baking paper to prevent it sticking to your worktop and roll it out to about ½ cm thickness.

Cut the dough into generous rounds or use autumn-themed cutters if you have them.

Place the rounds onto the prepared baking trays and chill in the fridge for at least 30 minutes to stop them spreading in the oven.

Bake for 20–25 minutes until the edges of your biscuits turn golden brown.

Sprinkle the tops of your shortbread with a little caster sugar mixed with a quarter of a teaspoon of autumn spice.

Allow to cool on the tray for 5 minutes then transfer to a wire rack.

Put the kettle on.

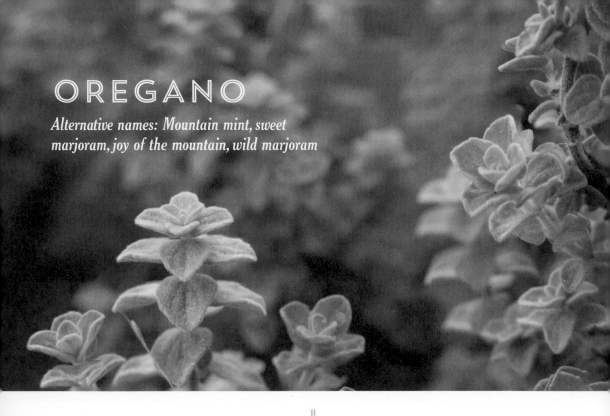

OREGANO

Alternative names: Mountain mint, sweet marjoram, joy of the mountain, wild marjoram

HOW TO IDENTIFY: Oregano's soft fuzzy olive-green leaves produce a slightly minty scent when crushed. The plant is topped with delicate purple flowers, which pollinators find very attractive when they blossom in the summer.

HISTORY: It was believed that oregano, which originated in Greece, was first grown by the goddess Aphrodite, who wanted it to be a symbol of joy in her garden.

The name oregano comes from the Greek words *"oros"*, meaning mountain, and *"ganos"*, meaning joy, "joy of the mountains", because it thrives on Mount Olympus and other Mediterranean mountain ranges.

The herb was soon popular for its taste, medicinal properties and ease of cultivation in Italy. Oregano was then transported all over Europe by the invading Roman army.

FOLKLORE: It was traditional for Greek brides and grooms to wear crowns of oregano woven together with laurel leaves to bring them happiness and joy in their married life.

Oregano can be used in spells for happiness, tranquillity, luck, health and protection. Oregano placed on the grave of a loved one also ensures that the deceased will find happiness in the afterlife.

Carry a sprig of oregano with you, decorate your house with it and grow it in your garden to protect yourself and your household from evil. A final rinse of oregano-infused water mopped onto your floor will cleanse your home and give you extra protection.

When worn on the head during sleep, oregano is said to promote psychic dreams. Rub olive oil infused with oregano onto bald patches to stimulate hair growth. Pop some oregano in your bathtub to help clear your thoughts and sprinkle dried oregano into your shoes to keep you safe during your travels.

FOLK MEDICINE: In medieval times, oregano was commonly used as a treatment for all manner of ailments, from coughing fits, toothache and indigestion to rheumatism and even melancholia.

Culpeper wrote that a powder of oregano mixed with honey soothes bruises; mixed with flour, oregano will treat inflamed eyes; and the *"juice dropped into the ears eases the pains and singing noises in them"*.

With antibiotic, antiviral and antifungal properties, oregano is a useful treatment for all sorts of common ailments such as athlete's foot and cold sores.

OTHER COMMON USES: Oregano is most often used in elements of Italian cooking, such as tomato sauces, as a pizza topping, in vegetable dishes and for adding flavour to grilled meat.

Oregano is a great substitute for marjoram or thyme if you don't have these in your spice cabinet.

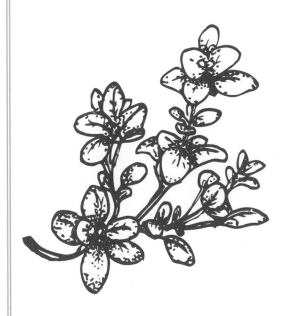

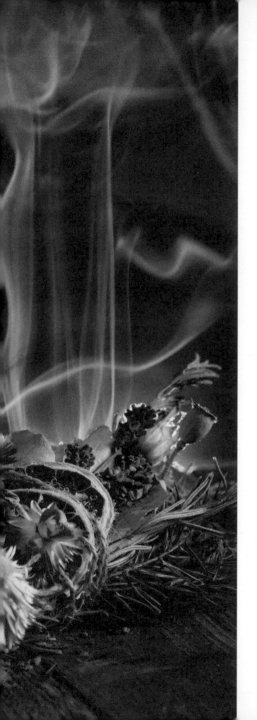

SMOULDER STICKS

You may have heard of bundles of white sage being used to "smudge" a dwelling; that is, to cleanse it of negative energy and prevent unwanted spirits from entering. Smudging is an ancient indigenous American cultural and spiritual practice, and the ritual burning of herbs is still performed all over the world to this day. The Celts carried out a very similar practice called "saining", which is the burning of herbal smoke with the intent to heal ailments or remove negative influences from people, places and animals.

As "smudging" and "saining" are very specific cultural names for a spiritual practice, I have decided, out of respect, to use the word "smoulder" for this activity.

Many different herbs and flowers can be made into smoulder sticks – in fact, anything that you have growing in your garden can be used depending on your intention, whether it be medicinal, cleansing or just to create pleasant smells.

Oregano is said to be a very effective cleansing herb. Folklore tells us that it will also help banish negativity and bring a sense of calm and happiness to the home.

My lovely sister-in-law Maria helped me make some gorgeous smoulder sticks using herbs and plants foraged from my garden. I think you'll agree that they are almost too beautiful to burn!

YOU WILL NEED:

Fresh herbs, flowers, greenery – choose items that you are attracted to

Natural twine

Other herbs to incorporate:

Lavender is calming

Lemongrass is energizing

Rose is peaceful

Rosemary enhances alertness and is a refreshing fragrance

Thyme is relaxing and uplifting

METHOD

Gather your ingredients. You'll need some longish stems to form a base. Rosemary, mugwort or lavender are good for this.

Put together your bunch of chosen herbs, just as if you are arranging a small bouquet. Make it look as pretty as you can.

Wrap the bunch up all the way up the stems with natural twine. The herbs will shrink as they dry and the twine may loosen, so bind them tightly.

Hang the bunches in a warm dry environment until they feel crispy and dry enough to burn. I tied mine on a branch in the shade of my big apple tree throughout the summer – remember to bring them in at night to avoid any dew or rain.

Once they feel completely dry, simply light one end and blow it out to make it smoulder.

After using your smoulder stick, douse it with plenty of water to ensure that it is out.

Only light outside or in a well-ventilated room away from curtains and animals.

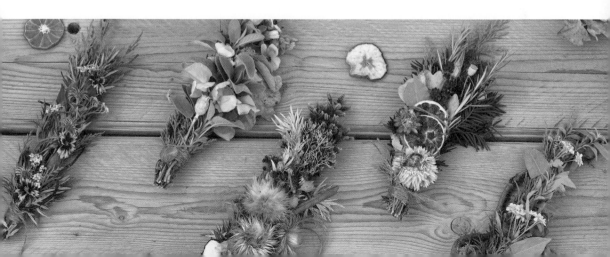

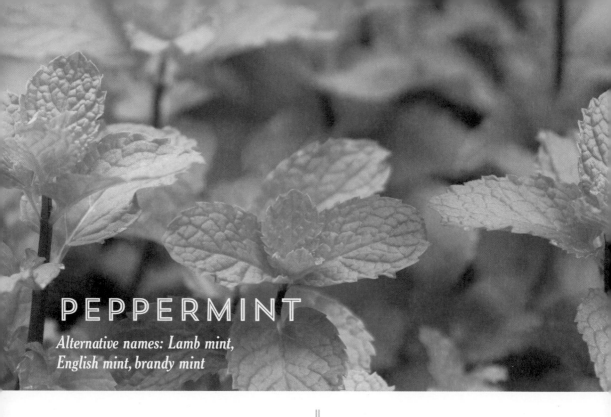

PEPPERMINT

Alternative names: Lamb mint,
English mint, brandy mint

HOW TO IDENTIFY: Peppermint is a hybrid between spearmint and watermint, with square stems, dark green leaves, clusters of pinkish flowers and a strong sweet scent.

HISTORY: There is evidence in Ancient Egyptian and Roman medical literature that peppermint was used to help ease stomach ailments and flatulence thousands of years ago.

First cultivated in Britain in the seventeenth century, peppermint was only used medicinally after it was published in the official list of medical drugs by the London Pharmacopoeia in 1721. Mitcham in Surrey became the centre of peppermint farming in Britain, where over 100 acres of land were devoted to the herb in the 1700s, expanding to 500 acres by 1850. The peppermint crop was transported to London, where it was distilled into essential oil for medicinal use, including a remedy for morning sickness, nausea and vomiting.

In the 1780s, the London-based confectioners Smith and Company invented

Altoids, "curiously strong" mints made from sugar, gum Arabic, oil of peppermint, gelatine and sucrose syrup. These mints would relieve "intestinal discomfort", with the added bonus that they also combatted bad breath.

FOLKLORE: Peppermint suspended over a sick bed will drive away negative energy and speed up healing, while polishing furniture and floorboards with peppermint oil will chase off any evil forces.

Smelling peppermint is believed to ease raw emotions, especially after a bereavement.

Place a few leaves in your purse or wallet to attract prosperity.

FOLK MEDICINE: Pliny the Elder believed that mint tea applied to the temples would ease a headache, while Greek physicians taught that it could prevent unwanted pregnancies and stop people vomiting blood.

Pliny prescribed mint powder to remove stomach parasites.

Both Culpeper and the herbalist John Gerard championed the use of mint for many ailments. In fact, Gerard proclaimed that mint was *"good against the watering eyes, and all manner of breakings out in the head, and against the infirmities of the fundament; it is a sure remedy for children's sore heads"*, and that it was *"a marvellous wholesome for the stomach"*.

OTHER COMMON USES: Peppermint essential oil is believed to be a deterrent to mice because they have a very keen sense of smell and find peppermint overwhelming and will stay away.

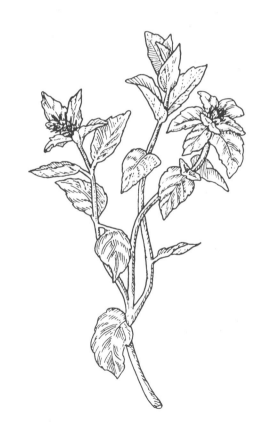

PEPPERMINT FOOT SCRUB

The wonderful cooling properties of peppermint make this foot scrub a real treat to use. Rosemary improves circulation and Epsom salts will exfoliate the skin to make your feet feel super soft.

INGREDIENTS

225 g Epsom salts or finely ground sea salt

100 ml carrier oil (try peach kernel, olive or sunflower)

1 tbsp fresh rosemary, finely chopped

10 drops peppermint essential oil

Equipment needed

Sterilized wide-mouthed jar

METHOD

Mix all the ingredients together thoroughly in a small bowl.

If you like your scrubs a little looser, add a bit more oil.

Pour the mixture into a wide-mouthed jar. Be aware that the oil will settle out and will need to be mixed in again before use.

This scrub is best used in a footbath with a towel to hand, because the oil will make your feet slippery.

Apply a scoop of scrub to each foot and massage in thoroughly – even better, get someone else to do it for you.

Rinse off and dry your feet.

Lasts approximately one year.

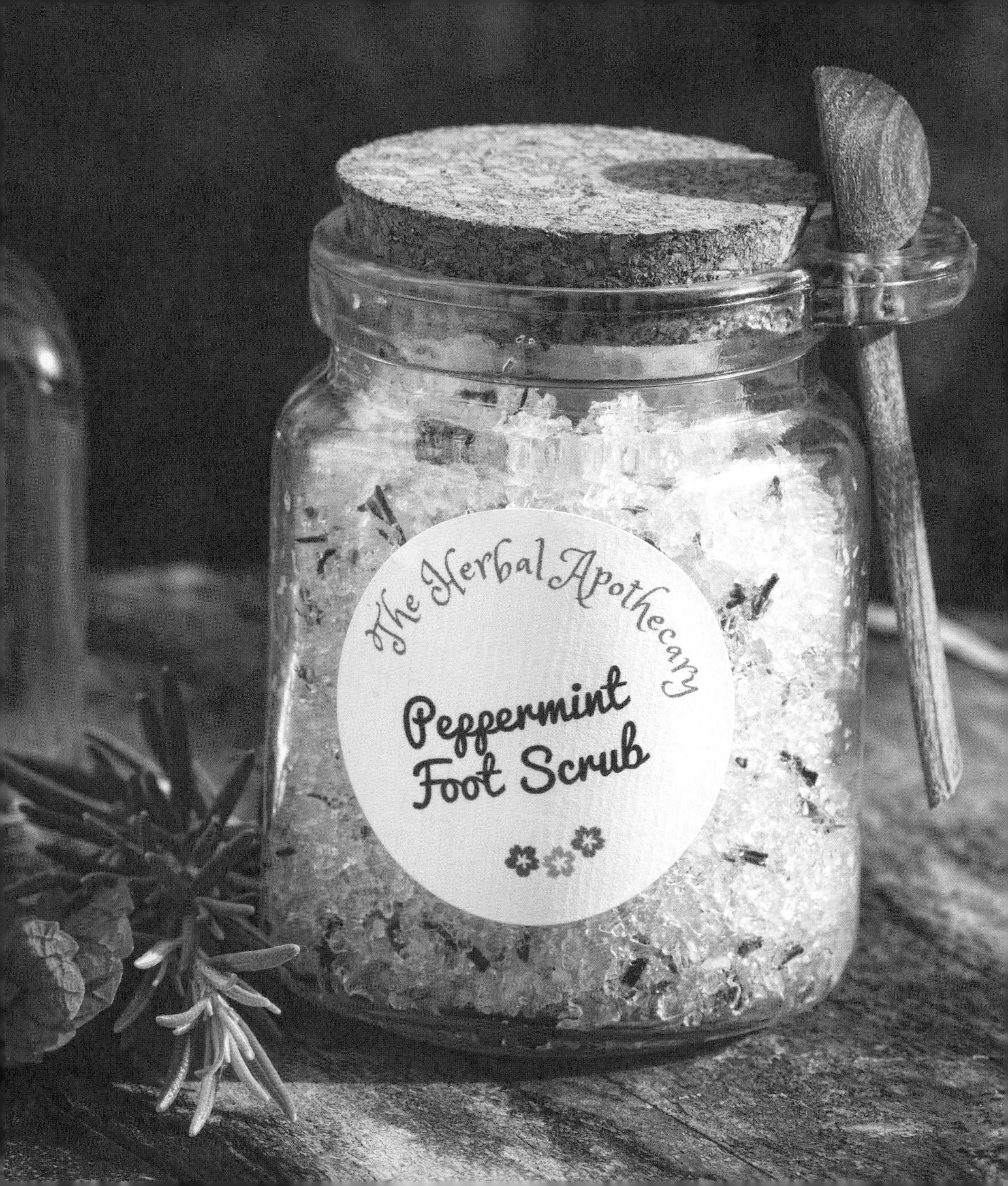
The Herbal Apothecary
Peppermint Foot Scrub

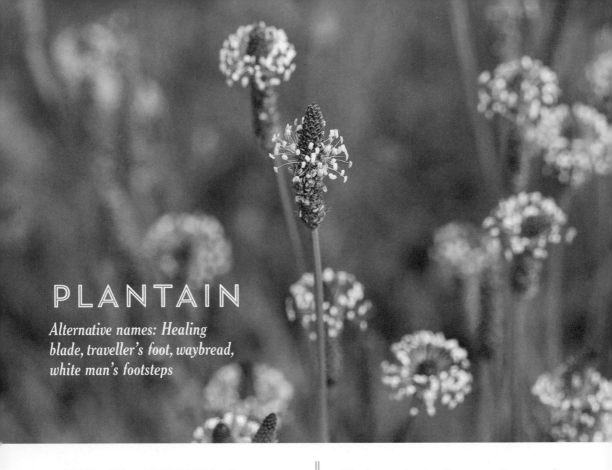

PLANTAIN

Alternative names: Healing blade, traveller's foot, waybread, white man's footsteps

HOW TO IDENTIFY: Plantain is a universal perennial plant found in lawns, at roadsides and on footpaths. Described by some as a short, fat, ugly weed, plantain is actually one of the best healing herbs on earth.

The broad, oval-shaped leaves grow in a rosette with distinctive stringy veins running from bottom to top.

The long, slender flower stalks grow from the central core, with many tiny greenish-yellow flowers that produce hundreds of seeds.

HISTORY: The plantain is often found growing alongside paths and tracks. As a result, it is trodden on frequently and seeds are picked up on the soles of shoes. The tough leaves lie flat and allow the herb to survive even the heaviest of trampling. Indigenous Americans gave plantain the name "white man's footsteps", precisely because the plant would self-seed wherever European settlers walked.

FOLKLORE: A necklace made from plantain will protect you from abduction by faeries, while an amulet made from plantain will protect you from insect stings and snake bites.

In the seventeenth century, English philosopher John Aubrey recalled how on the day of St John the Baptist, he witnessed a group of young women foraging, *"looking for the coal under the root of the plantain, to put under their bed at night, [so] they should dream of who would be their husbands".*

FOLK MEDICINE: Anglo-Saxon healers recited a "Nine Herbs Charm" to summon Odin the Norse god and therefore the ability to cure the sick. Plantain was included in the charm along with mugwort, lamb's cress, betony, camomile, nettle, crab apple, chervil and fennel. The herbs were pounded and made into a paste with ashes and egg and applied to wounds. Worn in the shoes, this mixture also eased the weariness of long-distance walkers and was believed to cure headaches when it was tied around the head with red cord.

In Shakespeare's *Love's Labour's Lost*, Costard calls for *"O, sir, plantain, a plain plantain!... no salve, sir, but a plantain!"* to mend his broken shin.

OTHER COMMON USES: Young leaves can be included in green salads, although they can be rather bitter. Still valuable as a traditional remedy for insect and nettle stings, the leaves are also antibacterial and anti-inflammatory. Chewing the leaves first makes this treatment more effective because it releases the active constituents needed for healing.

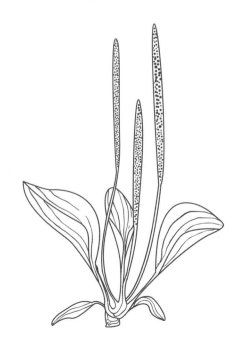

SPICED HOMEMADE AFTERSHAVE

As well as being easily recognizable and growing ubiquitously, plantain has lovely skin-soothing properties which make it perfect to include in this homemade aftershave recipe. Yarrow and witch hazel are added to help stop any bleeding from small shaving nicks and also to soothe razor burn.

This is a two-step process which takes a few weeks, so make sure to plan ahead, especially if you would like to make this as a gift.

SPICED RUM INFUSION

INGREDIENTS

A handful of fresh plantain leaves

3 tbsp fresh yarrow, chopped

8 cloves

1 large cinnamon stick broken into small pieces

¼ tsp ground allspice

125 ml white rum or vodka

Equipment needed

Sterilized jar

Piece of muslin

METHOD

Put the plantain, yarrow, cloves, cinnamon and allspice in a clean jar.

Cover the herbs and spices with rum, pop on a lid and shake.

Place the jar somewhere cool and dark for at least three weeks.

Strain the infused liquid through a muslin into a clean jar.

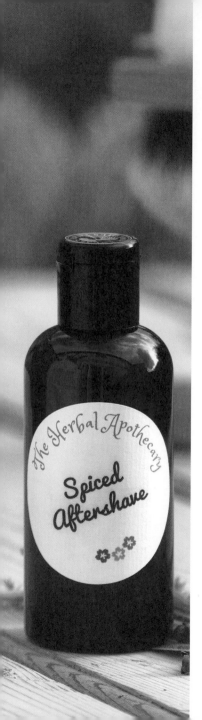

SPICED HOMEMADE AFTERSHAVE

INGREDIENTS

125 ml spiced rum infusion

Witch hazel

1 tbsp aloe vera gel
(see page 22)

10 drops black pepper
essential oil

3 drops sandalwood
essential oil

7 drops coriander
essential oil

Equipment needed

Glass jar or bottle

METHOD

It's important to dilute the spiced rum infusion to prevent stinging on freshly shaved skin. Start by adding 25 ml of witch hazel to your rum infusion along with the aloe vera in a glass jar or bottle; shake well.

Dab a little of the mixture onto the inside of your wrist. If the infusion makes your skin tingle or if the scent is too strong, add some more witch hazel to dilute the mixture.

Once you're happy with your dilution, add the essential oils and shake well.

Try it once again on your wrist to see if you are happy with the scent. Add a couple more drops of essential oils to increase the strength if desired.

Lasts approximately one year.

Always do a patch test.

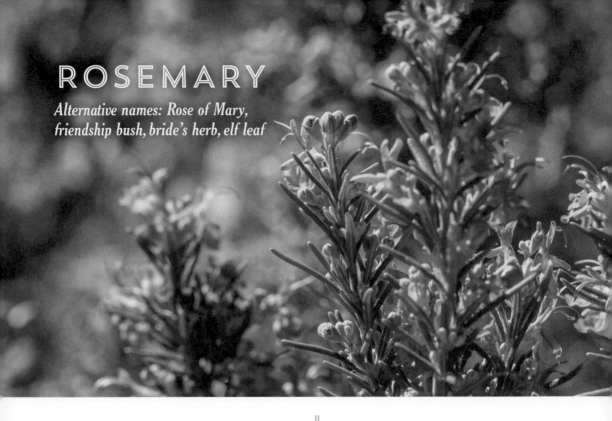

ROSEMARY

*Alternative names: Rose of Mary,
friendship bush, bride's herb, elf leaf*

HOW TO IDENTIFY: Rosemary is a tall fragrant bluish-grey herb with needle-like leaves and tiny blue flowers.

HISTORY: In the fourteenth century, Queen Philippa, the wife of King Edward III, received the first rosemary cuttings to come to Britain from her mother in Belgium. These were planted in the garden of the royal residence in the old palace of Westminster.

By the sixteenth century, its popularity had spread, and rosemary had become common in many gardens. John Parkinson, herbalist to Charles I, noted: *"not only that rosemary grows in every Englishwoman's Garden"*, but *"that it was commonly used as a token at both weddings and funerals"*. It was believed that rosemary in a bridal bouquet should then be planted in the garden of the newlyweds to be used at weddings of daughters and granddaughters.

Anne of Cleves carried rosemary in her wedding bouquet when she married Henry VIII, to symbolize love and fidelity. Unfortunately, this didn't really work for her – she was queen for just six months.

Rosemary was traditionally laid with the dead to disguise bad smells, and each mourner would throw a sprig into the coffin as a symbol of remembrance.

FOLKLORE: While fleeing to Egypt, the Virgin Mary laid her blue cloak over a white flowering rosemary bush to let it dry, turning the flowers blue forever. It is also believed that rosemary can only grow to the same height as Jesus and will only live to 33 years, Jesus' age at the time of his crucifixion.

Growing rosemary in your garden not only protects your family from witches but also ensures that you will never be short of friends. It grows particularly well in the garden of a dominant wife!

In the fourteenth century, the feet of thieves were washed in rosemary vinegar, supposedly to sap their energy and stop them from committing further crimes.

Hung over cradles, rosemary was said to protect babies from being stolen by faeries. Sniffed regularly, this herb will help you age gracefully. A man that doesn't love the smell of rosemary will never find true love.

FOLK MEDICINE: During the plague in the seventeenth century, rosemary was hung in houses and around the neck for protection from contagion. In London alone, 75,000 people died from the plague, making rosemary a very valuable commodity. In 1625, the price rose from 1 shilling (5 p) for an armful of rosemary branches to a whopping 6 shillings (30 p) for just a handful – bearing in mind that you could buy a whole pig for just 1 shilling (5 p), that does seem hugely expensive!

Rosemary was also burned along with juniper in hospitals and sick rooms to cleanse the air and stop the spread of infection.

OTHER COMMON USES: The smell of rosemary has been proven to stimulate the memory. Ancient Greek scholars would wear a sprig of rosemary when sitting exams to boost their performance – could be useful.

One of my absolute favourite culinary herbs, rosemary goes well with roast lamb, roasted Mediterranean vegetables and fish and chicken dishes.

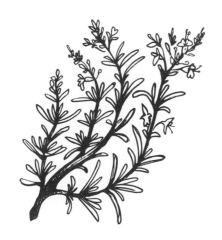

ROSEMARY BEARD OIL

This homemade rosemary beard oil moisturizes and softens coarse hair, making your beard look healthy and fuller. It also prevents itchiness and dandruff and may promote beard growth. This recipe is best made using dried rosemary, as fresh can sometimes make the oil go rancid.

INGREDIENTS

3 tbsp dried rosemary

100 ml carrier oil – jojoba is particularly good for beards

5 drops tea tree essential oil

5 drops sweet orange essential oil

Equipment needed

Sterilized jar

Piece of muslin

Dark glass bottle with dropper

METHOD

Put the rosemary into a clean, dry jar and pour over the carrier oil.

Put the lid on and place the jar on a sunny windowsill to infuse for at least four weeks.

The oil should have the aroma of rosemary. You can always add a little more and leave a while longer if you wish.

Once you are happy with the scent, filter the oil through a piece of muslin, giving it a good squeeze. Compost the rosemary if you can.

Add the essential oils and stir.

Decant into a suitable dark glass bottle with a dropper if you have one.

Store away from direct sunlight and this oil will last for approximately one year.

HOW TO USE:

Rub 3–5 drops of beard oil in the palms of your hands and massage it into your entire beard using downward strokes.

Work it thoroughly, combing through if necessary.

Always do a patch test.

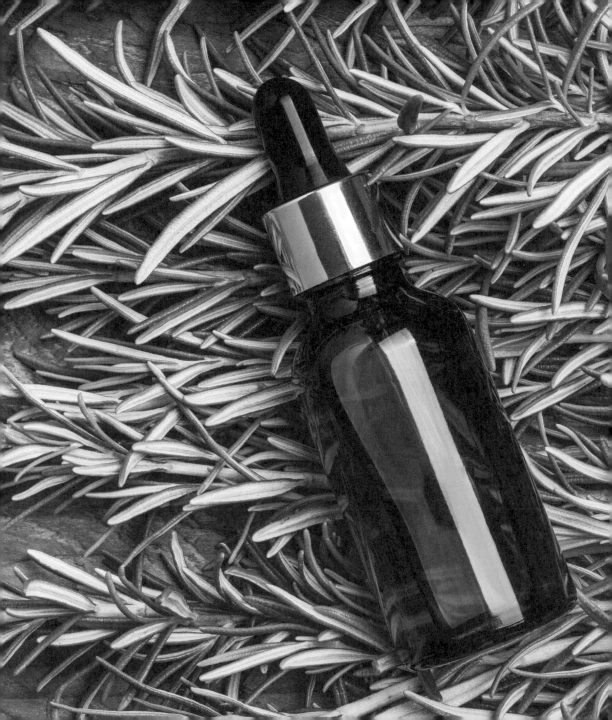

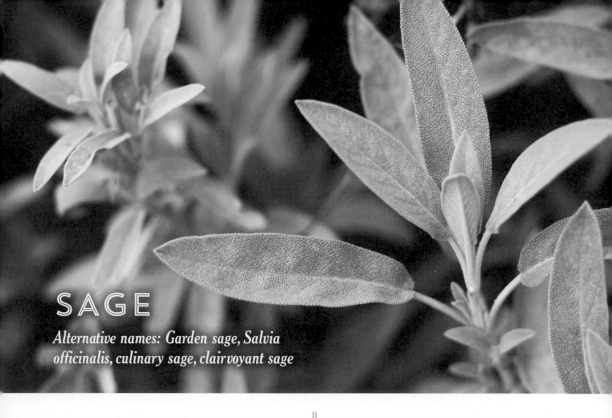

SAGE

Alternative names: Garden sage, Salvia officinalis, culinary sage, clairvoyant sage

HOW TO IDENTIFY: With soft, greyish green hairy leaves, this square-stemmed herb can grow up to 1.5 metres (5 feet) tall and can be identified by its distinctive strong earthy, musky smell.

HISTORY: Sage tea was drunk by Ancient Egyptian and Roman women to aid fertility. The Romans also used it to help them digest the fatty animal-based foods that made up a big part of their diet.

Like so many herbs that we rely on today, sage was introduced to Europe by the Romans. By the medieval period, sage was well established in apothecary gardens and monasteries around Europe.

FOLKLORE: In the medieval period, it was wise to look after the sage growing in your garden. If it flourished there, the fortunes and health of the household would prosper, too.

Like rosemary, it was believed that sage would grow well in the garden of a dominant woman – some men would cut the sage down rather than suffer the ridicule of friends and neighbours. In fact, J. A. Langford wrote in his nineteenth-century study of beliefs and superstitions local to Warwickshire that: *"If the sage tree thrives and grows, the master's not the master, and he knows."*

To manifest a wish, write it on a sage leaf, sleep with it under your pillow for three days and then bury it in your garden.

Carrying sage can make you wise (hence the name), and by eating it every day in May you will enjoy a long and healthy life.

The burning of different herbs has long been used in different cultures to cleanse, protect and purify houses, cattle and people. Smudging, which involves burning dry bundles of white sage to create a cleansing smoke, is used during exorcisms to drive out negative influences, bad spirits and to protect from evil.

FOLK MEDICINE: Many cures use sage for healthy teeth and gums. A traditional Romani toothpaste recipe from the 1940s consisted of equal parts chopped sage and salt and would be rubbed onto the teeth using Irish linen. A sage leaf with the vein removed can be put underneath dentures to relieve sore gums.

Sage was regarded as a cure-all by many. Culpeper recommended that *"leaves sodden in wine and laid upon the place affected with the palsy helps much, if the decoction be drank [...] helps the stinging and biting of serpents, and kills the worms that breed in the ear and in sores".*

OTHER COMMON USES: Sage and onion stuffing not only tastes great but will help you digest your Sunday lunch, too!

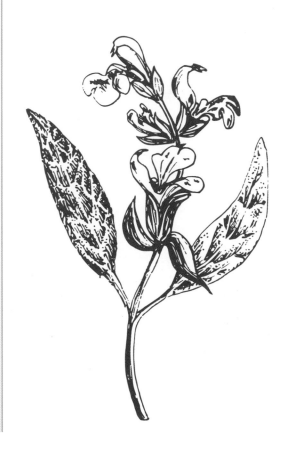

AROMATIC FIRESTARTERS

This is a great way to use up all the odds and ends of candles that are too small to burn. Check your cupboards for out-of-date dried herbs and use those up, too. These firestarters can be used to light campfires, fire pits and open fires but *not* gas burning stoves or wood burners. Use with caution in all cases.

YOU WILL NEED

Candle ends, soy wax or beeswax

Twine, cut into approximately 5-cm lengths

Cupcake cases, empty egg boxes or dry pinecones

A selection of dried or fresh herbs such as sage, thyme, rosemary, bay leaves

METHOD

Carefully melt all the candle ends together in a double boiler placed over hot water.

Dip your piece of twine in the melted wax to form a wick and then nestle it into each cupcake case or egg box section.

Pour melted wax on top of the wick until each firestarter paper case is half full. If you are using cupcake cases, use the support of a cupcake tray.

While the wax is still soft, poke in fresh bundles of herbs, cinnamon sticks, dried citrus slices and scatter with dried herbs.

Allow the firestarters to cool completely and then store in an airtight tin.

To use, place one cupcake firestarter or two egg box sections into the grate with kindling and paper and light the wick.

Dry foraged pinecones also make lovely firestarters. Simply dip the cones in the melted wax, add the herbs or essential oils of your choice then snuggle them among your kindling.

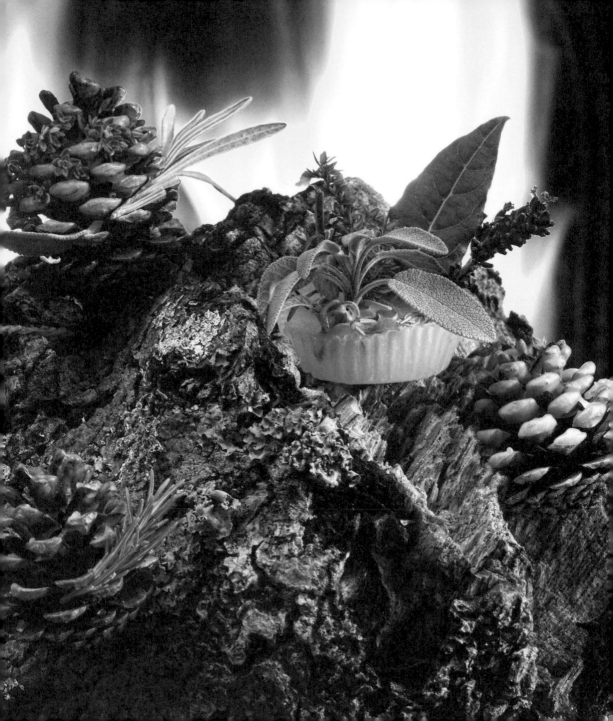

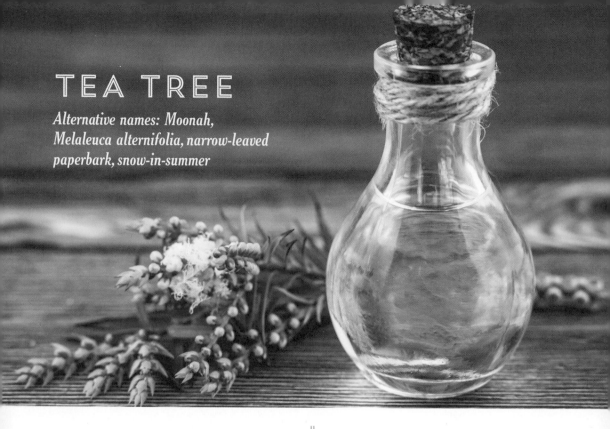

TEA TREE

Alternative names: Moonah,
Melaleuca alternifolia, narrow-leaved
paperbark, snow-in-summer

HOW TO IDENTIFY: This evergreen tree can grow to around 7 metres (20 feet) tall with smooth narrow leaves and small white flowers forming a bottle-brush shape.

HISTORY: Known to the indigenous Aborigines of Australia for thousands of years, tea tree leaves were chewed to ease headaches and used to make antifungal and antiseptic poultices by combining crushed leaves and mud. The bark, which was soft and pliable, was used as a bandage, a sleeping mat, a liner for babies' cots and as a building material.

The medicinal properties of this wonderful plant were completely unknown outside aboriginal culture until the 1920s, when an Australian chemist, Dr Arthur Penfold, began to research the antiseptic properties of tea tree. Penfold published a scientific paper in 1929 revealing that the antiseptic powers of tea tree were 12 times that of carbolic acid, the accepted antiseptic at that time.

A flurry of research followed, and tea tree essential oil was included in the first aid kits of the Australian armed forces during the Second World War. Producers of tea tree oil were exempt from being called up to fight to ensure that there was enough of this healing oil to be sent out to hospitals and for first aid kits.

FOLKLORE: The Bunurong people of Australia have a legend of the sacred Moonah (tea tree), which was borne out of forbidden love. A young Bunurong couple had fallen madly in love and spent all their time tightly embraced in each other's arms instead of carrying out their daily duties. The village elders warned the couple that they should not forget their responsibilities and must help with the day-to-day work. This warning was ignored, and the couple were banished from their people – but this did nothing to break their relationship. They continued with their tight embraces until they eventually froze in place, their entwined bodies becoming the twisted trunk and branches of the Moonah tree. Their love spread and they covered the island with their children, who still grow there today.

FOLK MEDICINE: Aborigines used to crush the leaves and extract the oil, which was then inhaled as a decongestant to treat colds and coughs.

Tea tree essential oil can be used topically for insect bites, skin infections and general healing of the skin. Its antibacterial, antifungal and anti-inflammatory properties can be used to repel insects, treat athlete's foot, combat body odour and treat dandruff.

OTHER COMMON USES: Tea tree can be used to make a natural all-purpose disinfectant cleaning spray. Combine 20 drops of tea tree essential oil with 500 ml water in a spray bottle, shake well. Spray directly onto surfaces and wipe with a clean cloth.

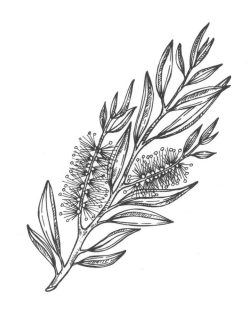

TEA TREE AND ROSEMARY SHOWER STEAMERS

Tea tree essential oil fights infection, boosts immunity and helps ease the symptoms of coughs and colds. Rosemary is a great essential oil to get your brain going first thing in the morning because it encourages mental alertness and focus – something you really need if you are suffering from a cold!

Combine these two essential oils together in a shower steamer and get your day off to a really good start.

INGREDIENTS

100 g bicarbonate of soda

50 g citric acid

50 g cornflour or arrowroot powder

20 drops tea tree essential oil

20 drops rosemary essential oil

Witch hazel in a spray bottle

Equipment needed

Silicone moulds, ice cube trays or cupcake cases

Rubber gloves

METHOD

Combine all the dry ingredients and mix with a fork or a whisk to break up any lumps.

Add the essential oils and whisk again.

Pop on your rubber gloves as some of the ingredients may irritate sensitive skin. Spray a small amount of witch hazel onto the dry ingredients and mix with your hands. Don't add too much witch hazel or the mixture will begin to fizz.

The mixture should feel like wet sand and hold together when squeezed.

Press firmly into your moulds.

Leave to dry for 24–48 hours, until the steamers feel hard and set.

Gently push them out of the moulds and store in an airtight jar.

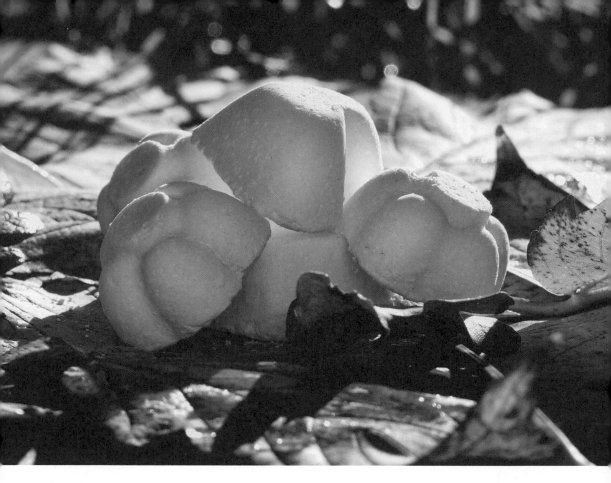

TO USE

Place a shower steamer into your shower tray, step inside and enjoy the delicious aromas released as it fizzes under the running water.

Try making steamers with a combination of your favourite essential oils to enjoy when you don't have a cold.

Always do a patch test.

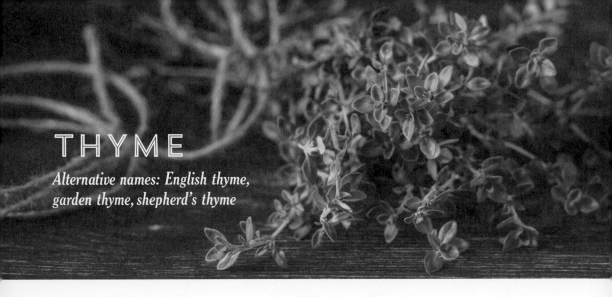

THYME

Alternative names: English thyme, garden thyme, shepherd's thyme

HOW TO IDENTIFY: Thyme is a low-growing woody herb with small aromatic leaves growing all the way up the stems.

HISTORY: Wild thyme is one of Britain's native species and can still be found there growing on heathland and in meadows. The many other varieties of thyme, such as lemon thyme and creeping thyme, originated in Mediterranean regions and were spread far and wide by the Romans.

Along with other fragrant herbs, thyme was rubbed into the bodies of the Egyptian pharaohs as part of the mummification process; it was also believed to ease the passage of the spirit into the afterlife.

It was believed that eating thyme and even bathing in thyme would give protection from poisoning; this made it especially popular with understandably nervous Roman emperors.

Thyme was burned in both Roman and Greek temples for purification. Inhaling the smoke was also believed to give courage to soldiers about to go into battle.

FOLKLORE: Faeries love to inhabit the twisted and knotted branches of wild thyme. It is therefore unlucky to bring thyme into the home because you can run the risk of upsetting the fae. However, thyme can be sprinkled on windowsills and doorsteps should you wish to invite the faery folk to visit, and bathing your eyes in the dew from thyme leaves before dawn on the first day of May will enable you to see your special visitors. Patches of wild thyme were evidence that faeries had partied the night away on that very spot – this led to generations of young girls camping out in the hope of glimpsing faeries. To find a lost object, leave an offering of thyme and honey in the woods on the night of a full moon and the faeries will do their best to find it for you.

Roma will never bring wild thyme into their wagons, regarding it as unlucky. They will, however, drink thyme tea outdoors with a little vinegar and honey to cure a cough.

Plant thyme at the beginning of the waxing moon with several coins tucked into the root ball. Look after it well and as the thyme grows so will your bank balance.

FOLK MEDICINE: Plague doctors in fourteenth-century England believed that diseases were carried by "miasma" (bad air), so they wore long beak-like masks stuffed with many herbs including thyme, peppermint and rosemary to avoid becoming infected by their patients.

To quote Culpeper:

"[Thyme] purges the body of phlegm, and is an excellent remedy for shortness of breath. It kills worms in the belly [...] gives safe and speedy delivery to women in travail [labour] and brings away the afterbirth."

Thyme is a natural antiseptic and antibiotic and has been used to treat a myriad of ailments including coughs, colds, warts, sciatica, headaches, hay fever and hangovers. Even before bacteria and infection were properly understood, nurses in the nineteenth century were soaking bandages in a solution of thyme water.

OTHER COMMON USES: Thymol is the powerful antiseptic contained in thyme. It can be found in mouthwash, hand sanitizer and acne cream.

Bees love flowering thyme, and the resulting honey takes on a delicious herby flavour that is much sought after by honey lovers.

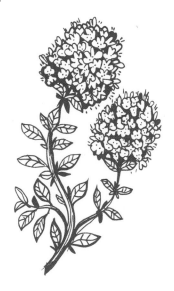

HERBAL FACIAL STEAM

Herbal steams have long been used to cleanse and soothe skin, give relief from headaches and nasal congestion and to promote good circulation.

Herbs can be chosen according to what it is you wish to achieve. For brightening dull winter skin, choose calendula, lavender and lemon balm. For irritated skin, camomile is best. Camomile, lavender, rose and fennel are best for dry skin, and peppermint, sage, lavender and camomile are best for oily skin.

Thyme is an expectorant, meaning that it will help to loosen and clear phlegm from blocked noses and sinuses. It is also very gentle and doesn't irritate the skin.

Makes enough for one steam treatment

INGREDIENTS

1 tbsp dried thyme or a good sprig of fresh

1 tbsp dried sage or a good sprig of fresh

1 tbsp dried rosemary or a good sprig of fresh

500 ml just-boiled water

5 drops eucalyptus essential oil

Equipment needed

Heatproof bowl

Clean towel

METHOD

Create a space where you can safely use boiling water – a kitchen table will do.

Put the herbs into a heatproof bowl and cover with 500 ml of just-boiled water.

Add the eucalyptus essential oil.

Create a tent with a towel that covers your head and the bowl. Don't put your face too close to the steam to avoid burning your skin.

Inhale deeply for 10–15 minutes.

Repeat as needed.

Steaming is not recommended if you have sensitive or sunburned skin.

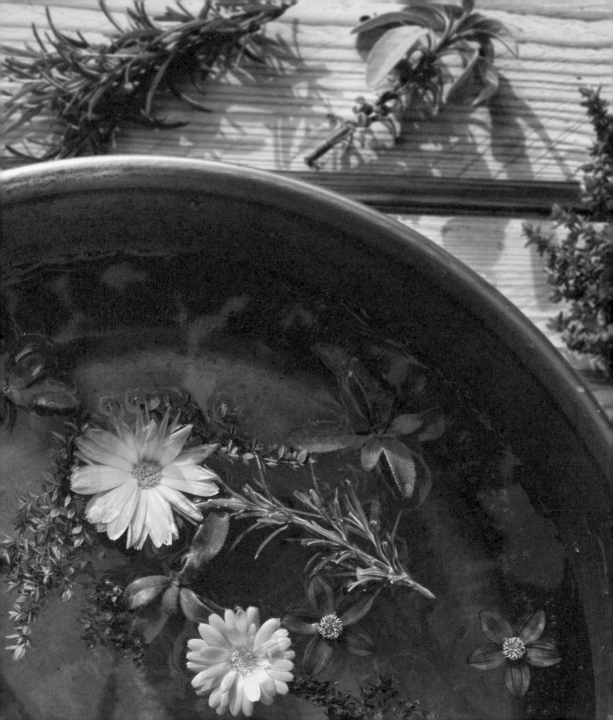

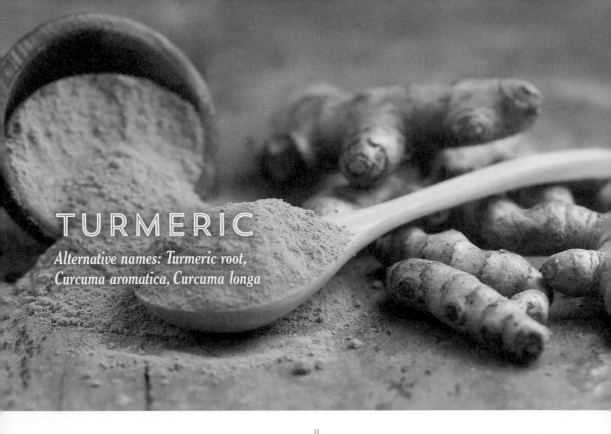

TURMERIC

*Alternative names: Turmeric root,
Curcuma aromatica, Curcuma longa*

HOW TO IDENTIFY: Turmeric is the vivid golden orange fragrant spice which comes from the underground stems (rhizomes) of the turmeric plant. Turmeric thrives in moist tropical climates because the rhizomes prefer light well-drained soil. In the right conditions, the plant can reach up to a metre (3 feet) high. With long simple leaves, turmeric produces yellow-white flowers on a spike-like stalk.

Turmeric root is available fresh but is much more familiar in its dried and powdered form.

HISTORY: Native to China, southern India, Indonesia and the islands of the Indian Ocean, turmeric has been cultivated for more than 2,000 years for use as a condiment, vegetable dye, medicine, perfume and in cosmetics.

Turmeric is thought to have been brought to Europe in the thirteenth century by merchants such as Marco Polo, who in his notes recorded *"there is a vegetable that has all the properties of true saffron, as well as the smell and the colour and yet is not really saffron".*

In medieval Europe, turmeric was known as "Indian saffron", and, because of its high price, was flaunted as a status symbol by the wealthy.

FOLKLORE: In Indian culture, turmeric, known as *"haldi"*, has a particularly important role in Hindu weddings and even has a whole ceremony named after it! On the day before their wedding, the bride and groom are covered in a paste made from turmeric by the female members of the house. If any unmarried friends are touched by the paste, they will soon be married, too. It is believed that the Haldi ceremony will protect the couple from evil spirits, ensure prosperity, purify, cleanse and balance the energies of their bodies, relieve wedding-day nerves and bless the couple with a very happy married life.

FOLK MEDICINE: Culpeper wrote in his *Complete Herbal* that *"rosemary, saffron and turmeric root infused in rhenish [German] wine, is a cure for the jaundice, and brings down the menses [menstruation]"*.

In Indian Ayurvedic holistic medicine, turmeric is burned and inhaled to ease congestion. It is also made into a paste to treat shingles and blemishes and to counteract the ageing process. As a result, turmeric is known as *"matrimanika"*, meaning "as beautiful as moonlight".

OTHER COMMON USES: Due to the high cost of saffron, turmeric was used as an alternative to dye cloth a beautiful sunshine gold colour.

Turmeric can also be used as a natural indicator of pH. When mixed with an acidic solution it will turn yellow, but it will turn red if the solution is alkaline.

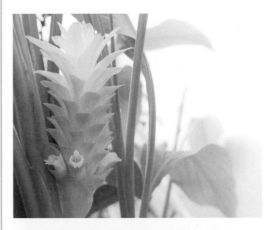

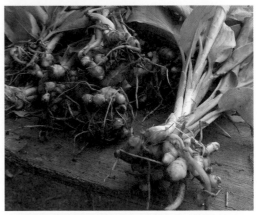

INDIAN GOLDEN MILK (HALDI DOODH)

Research has discovered that turmeric has antioxidant, anti-inflammatory, antibacterial and antifungal properties. Black pepper contains piperine, which helps our bodies to absorb more curcumin, the active ingredient in turmeric that helps the body to reduce inflammation. Cardamom seeds, clove buds and ginger all have antioxidant and antibacterial properties to help boost the immune system.

This golden milk recipe has long been used to ease many ailments, from coughs and colds to inflammation and aches and pains. It's a very comforting brew and can be made with whatever milk you prefer; I especially like making it with almond milk, but cow's milk works well, too.

One word of warning: turmeric stains everything it touches!

Serves two

INGREDIENTS

2–3 cm fresh turmeric

1 cm fresh ginger

500 ml milk (animal or plant based)

4 black peppercorns

Seeds from 2 cardamom pods

2 clove buds

Honey or maple syrup to sweeten

METHOD

Finely grate the turmeric and ginger into a small saucepan with the milk, no need to peel.

Crush the peppercorns, cardamom pods and clove buds and add to the pan along with the turmeric, ginger and milk.

Bring to a gentle boil, stir and remove from the heat.

Cover the pan and allow to steep for 5 minutes.

Pour the mixture through a sieve into two small cups and sweeten to taste.

Enjoy.

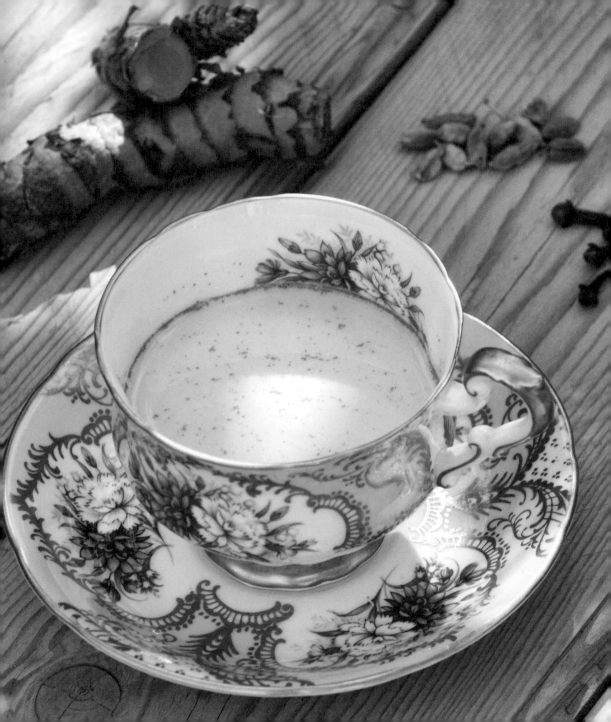

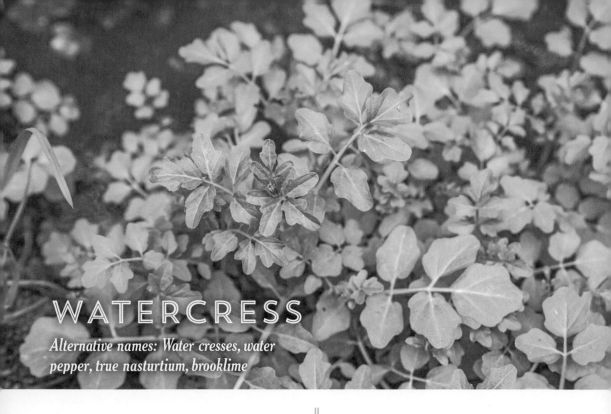

WATERCRESS

Alternative names: Water cresses, water pepper, true nasturtium, brooklime

HOW TO IDENTIFY: Growing in cool running water, watercress is a hot and peppery fast-growing herb with small white flowers.

HISTORY: The Greek physician Hippocrates chose to found a hospital on the island of Kos so that he could use the natural springs to grow the watercress he would need to treat blood disorders.

Greek, Roman and Persian soldiers, as well as children, were fed a daily diet of watercress when it was observed that people enjoyed better physical health when they ate the herb. It was usually served as a salad with oil and vinegar, pepper, cumin and lentiscus (mastic leaves).

In 1800s Britain, watercress sandwiches were a staple part of the diet of the working classes, mainly because the plant could be picked for free from rivers and streams. The health benefits of watercress made it very popular, and the Hampshire town of Alresford soon became the centre of the watercress industry. The establishment of the watercress train line in 1865 meant that the produce could be transported to London while it was still fresh.

Street vendors, usually children, would sell posies of watercress at Covent Garden market. The herb was often eaten in a sandwich for breakfast, known as "the poor man's bread".

The austerity measures caused by two world wars led to the gradual decline of the watercress line, and its closure in the 1960s signalled the end for many growers as they couldn't easily get their produce to market. However, watercress is still grown in Hampshire and West Sussex and is gaining in popularity as we all try to make healthier choices and support local producers.

FOLKLORE: Legend has it that Gall, the ancient king of Ulster, was cured of his "madness" when he drank the water and ate watercress from the holy well near Dingle in County Kerry. In Scotland and Ireland, it was believed that when placed in the pail, watercress could take all the goodness out of milk.

Burning watercress will drive away snakes. If you pop some under your bed, the smell will help to create a little passion in the bedroom.

FOLK MEDICINE: Nicholas Culpeper recommended a decoction of watercress to cure ulcers and wrote that it could be applied to the face overnight and then rinsed away to remove any blemishes. Watercress juice is also *very good for those that are dull or drowsy, or have lethargy*.

OTHER COMMON USES: Watercress is best eaten raw to preserve all the wonderful nutrients. It adds a peppery hit to salads, smoothies, pesto, sandwiches and dips.

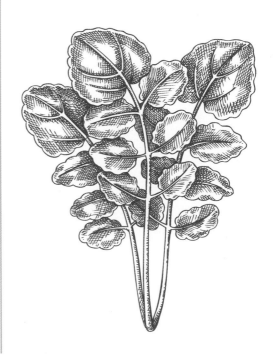

WATERCRESS HUMMUS

This superfood is high in iron, potassium, calcium, vitamins A and C, as well as antioxidants. Adding watercress to this hummus recipe will give you all the benefits in a quick and healthy dip that is delicious on its own or spread on wraps or crackers.

INGREDIENTS

400 g can of chickpeas, drained (save the liquid)

50 g watercress

1 garlic clove finely chopped

3 tbsp olive oil

1 tbsp tahini paste

Lemon juice to taste

Salt and pepper

Equipment needed

Stick blender

METHOD

Use a stick blender to combine all the ingredients except the lemon juice and salt and pepper.

Add enough chickpea water to make a smooth paste.

Add a squeeze of lemon and season to taste.

Keep in the fridge and consume within three days.

AUTHOR'S CHEAT: Short of time? Buy a tub of plain hummus and some watercress and whizz the two together.

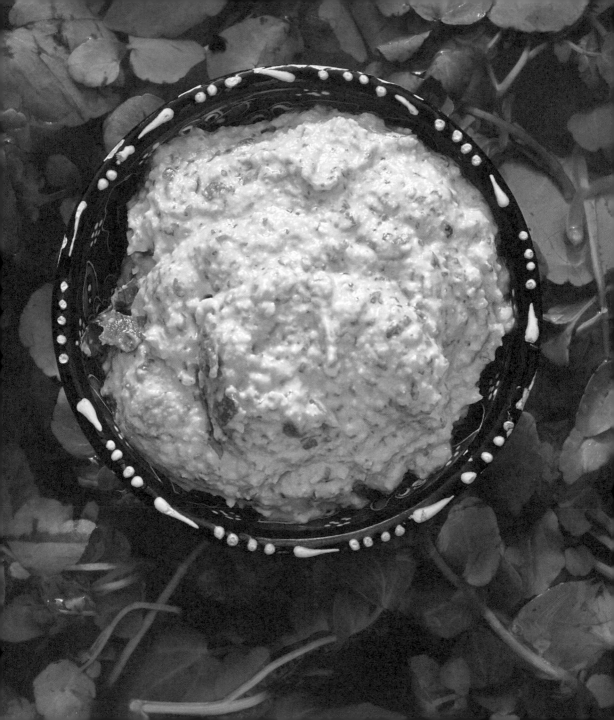

WITCH HAZEL

Alternative names: Spotted alder, winterbloom, snapping hazelnut, tobacco wood

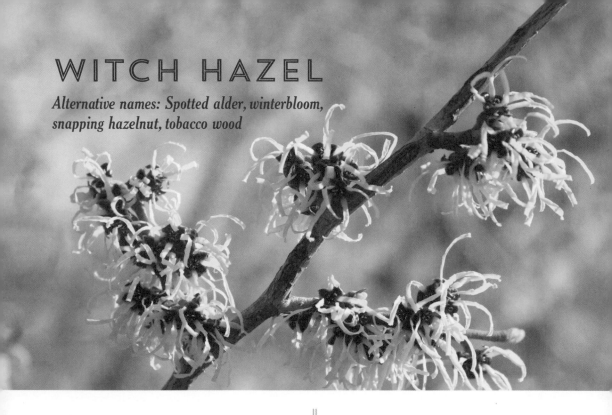

HOW TO IDENTIFY: This flowering shrub is most recognizable by its yellow spider-like flowers, which bloom on bare branches in the autumn.

HISTORY: The name witch hazel doesn't actually have anything to do with witches! It is believed to come from the old English *"wice"*, *"wicke"* or *"wiche"*, meaning bendable or pliant.

European settlers were shown how to use witch hazel sticks to dowse for underground water by the indigenous American Mohegan tribe. In the 1950s, the American botanist Donald Peattie wrote in *A Natural History of North American Trees* that naturally Y-shaped branches would be chosen, those *"whose points grew north and south so that they had the influence of the sun at its rising and setting, and you carried it with a point in each hand, the stem pointing forward. Any downward tug of the stem was caused by the flow of hidden water"*.

Witch hazel was one of the first plants chosen for ornamental use in private botanical gardens as early as the seventeenth century, but it isn't clear exactly who brought it to Britain. By the eighteenth century, it was one of many American plants that had become fashionable among British garden circles.

In 1846, pharmacist Theron T. Pond learned about the benefits of distilled witch hazel extract from indigenous Americans living around New York. He went on to use it as an ingredient in Pond's cold cream and to establish a very successful cosmetics company.

FOLKLORE: Many modern witches consider witch hazel a magical herb and use it to heal broken hearts. Some believe tea made from witch hazel leaves and bark will heighten occult powers, while amulets made from witch hazel wood can be carried as protection against evil spirits.

FOLK MEDICINE: The Osage tribe of North America use witch hazel bark to treat sores and skin ulcers. The Iroquois brew a tea to treat coughs, colds and dysentery, and the Potawatomi steam the twigs over hot rocks in their sweat lodges to soothe sore muscles.

In the 1830s, an astringent ointment for haemorrhoids could be purchased in pharmacies consisting of equal parts witch hazel, white oak and sweet apple bark.

OTHER COMMON USES: Because of its natural astringent properties, witch hazel is still in use for many minor skin ailments; it eases razor burn after shaving, speeds up the healing of bruises, soothes eczema, cools sunburn, reduces itching from insect bites and even eases the itching and pain from haemorrhoids.

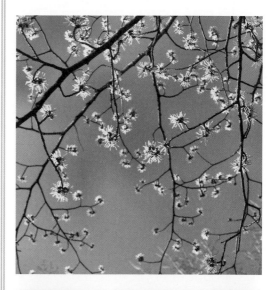

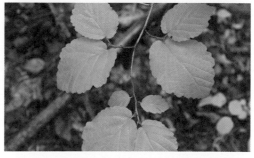

WITCH HAZEL DEODORANT

Distilled from the bark and twigs, witch hazel water is a tried-and-tested skin friendly ingredient and is widely available in chemists. Clove oil calms irritated skin, coriander oil has deodorizing properties, lavender oil is anti-inflammatory, lemon and lime oils reduce body odour and palmarosa oil is antibacterial – combined, this homemade deodorant smells amazing!

INGREDIENTS

90 ml distilled witch hazel

10 ml vegetable glycerine

2 drops clove essential oil

2 drops coriander essential oil

2 drops lavender oil

10 drops lemon essential oil

5 drops lime essential oil

5 drops palmarosa essential oil

Equipment needed

Sterilized 100-ml bottle fitted with an atomizer spray

METHOD

Mix all ingredients together in a small jug and pour into the bottle.

Tightly screw on the atomizer lid and shake well before use.

Will keep for up to six months.

Always do a patch test.

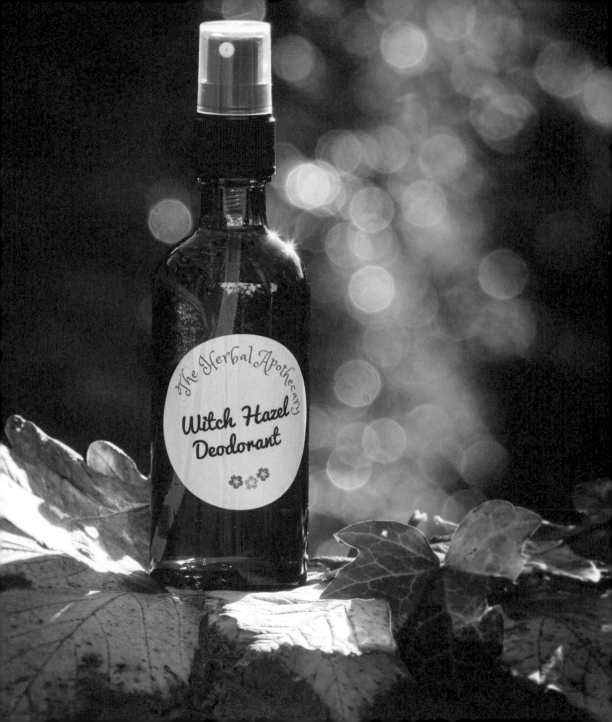

The Herbal Apothecary

Witch Hazel
Deodorant

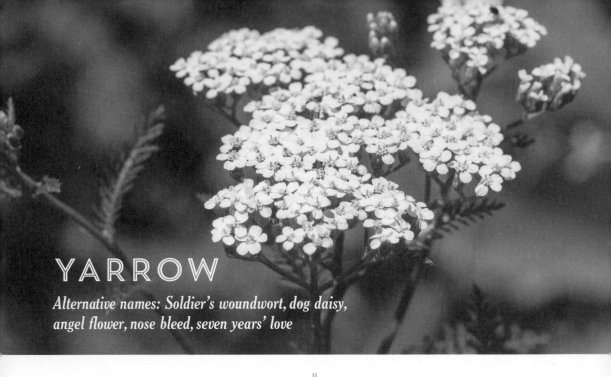

YARROW

*Alternative names: Soldier's woundwort, dog daisy,
angel flower, nose bleed, seven years' love*

HOW TO IDENTIFY: Yarrow is found in abundance in grassland all over Britain. This ferny leafed perennial can grow up to 1 metre (3 feet) tall. The plant has long, straight stalks and feathery leaves with pink or white flowers at the top. It forms clumps that can be quite invasive. Crush the leaves and you will release its strong aromatic smell.

HISTORY: The Anglo-Saxons had great respect for yarrow due to its powerful wound-healing properties.

In the medieval period, before the widespread use of hops, yarrow was one of the many herbs, along with bog myrtle and wild rosemary, used to make "gruit", an early form of beer.

FOLKLORE: Unmarried maidens in medieval Sussex would pick yarrow from a young man's grave by the light of the full moon and put it under their pillow, saying:

> *"Goodnight fair yarrow,*
> *Thrice goodnight to thee,*
> *I hope before tomorrow,*
> *My true love to see."*

When they got home, the yarrow was placed in a drawer; if it was still fresh the next morning, their love would be reciprocated. They would also pin it to their dresses and get as close to their potential suitor as possible.

Often known as "seven years' love", yarrow was included in bridal bouquets, hung over the marriage bed and often eaten at wedding breakfasts to ensure that the couple were happy for at least seven years.

FOLK MEDICINE: Yarrow has been used as a remedy for many ailments. The dark blue essential oil from the flowers is a good chest rub for colds and flu.

Leaves, stems and flowers are used to lower blood pressure and help maintain healthy circulation.

An infusion of yarrow applied to the scalp will prevent baldness but unfortunately won't be able to cure it. Headaches were believed to be caused by too much blood pressure in the head and yarrow leaves were pushed up the nostrils to cause bleeding that would ease the pressure. According to John Gerard, in his *The Herball or Generall Historie of Plants* (1597): *"The leaves being put into the nose do cause it to bleed, and easeth the pain of megrin [migraine]."* Conversely, smelling yarrow flowers was believed to be a cure for nosebleeds because the leaves encourage clotting.

If you were unfortunate enough to become infected by the plague, there were many remedies that Markham could recommend, including: *"Take yarrow, tansy, feverfew, of each a handful, and bruise them well together, then let the sick party make water into the herbs, then strain them, and give it to the sick to drink."*

OTHER COMMON USES: Yarrow is a very useful herb to hang in your wardrobe because it deters moths and other insects. Yarrow was a popular vegetable in the seventeenth century when the young leaves were cooked like spinach or put into soup. The leaves can also be dried and used as a cooking herb.

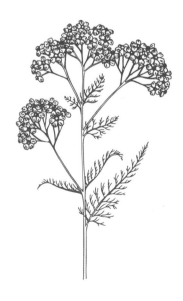

YARROW AND ROSEMARY HERBAL RINSE FOR HAIR

Herbal hair rinses are simple to make and can increase hair's body and shine, as well as enhancing natural high- and lowlights. Yarrow has antiseptic, anti-inflammatory and astringent properties that can ease the symptoms of dandruff and help manage greasy hair.

Makes one application

INGREDIENTS

2 tbsp dried yarrow

1 tbsp dried rosemary

500 ml filtered water, boiled

Equipment needed

Heatproof jug

Piece of muslin

METHOD

Put the dried herbs in a heatproof jug and pour over the boiled water.

Cover and leave to steep overnight or for at least 8 hours.

Strain the herbs from the liquid through a muslin cloth into a jug, squeezing to get out every last drop. Compost the herbs if you can.

HOW TO USE

Wash your hair as normal.

Pour some herbal rinse over your hair, catching as much of the liquid in the jug as you can so that you can rinse several times.

Massage the infusion well into scalp and hair, avoiding your eyes.

Reapply several times and do not rinse out.

This herbal rinse is best made fresh every time you wish to use it.

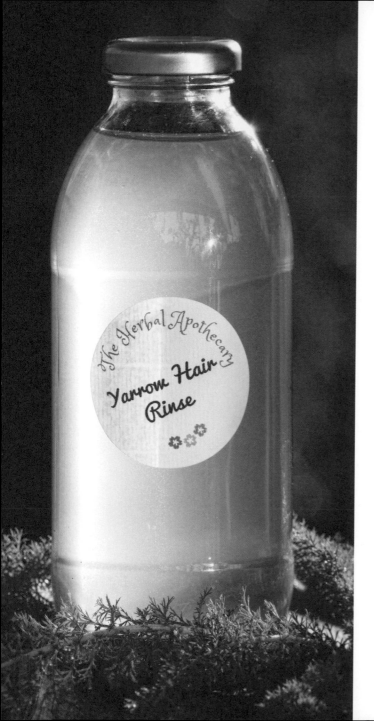

OTHER HERBS TO TRY

FOR DRY HAIR: calendula, camomile, lavender, nettle, sage

FOR THINNING HAIR: sage, nettle, rosemary, basil

FOR DARK HIGHLIGHTS: rosemary, sage, black tea, nettle

FOR RED HIGHLIGHTS: red rose petals, calendula, hibiscus flowers, red clover flowers

FOR GOLDEN HIGHLIGHTS: camomile, sunflower petals, calendula

FOR OILY HAIR: yarrow, peppermint, lemon balm, thyme

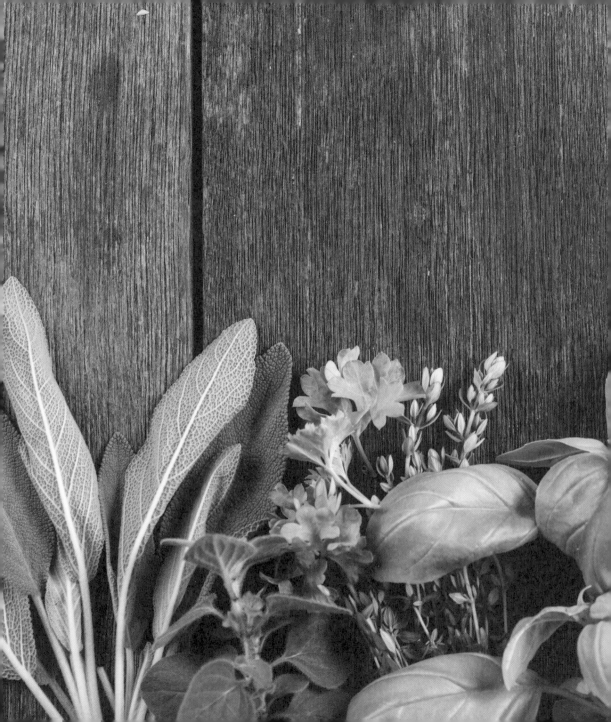

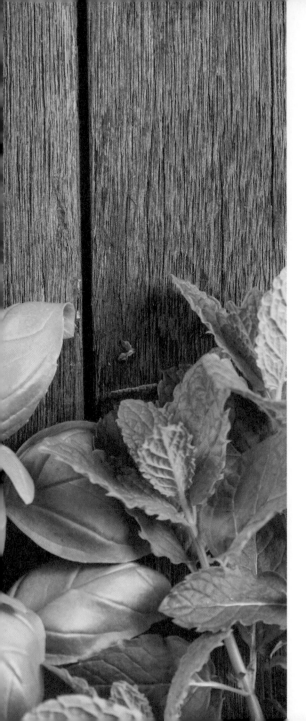

FINAL THOUGHTS

My interest in the fascinating folklore and healing properties of plants began with *The Hedgerow Apothecary*, expanded into *The Garden Apothecary* and now I have been on a whole new voyage of personal discovery with my latest book, *The Herbal Apothecary* – and what a wonderful journey it has been!

I have followed the path taken by ancient merchants learning some wonderful traditions, made fascinating discoveries about other cultures and gained a newfound appreciation of what I take very much for granted in my spice rack. Our lives and our kitchens have been so enriched by these incredible herbs and spices; it's hard to imagine a time when we didn't have them – cookery must have been very bland indeed.

I hope that you've enjoyed the journey with me.

ONLINE SUPPLIERS

G. Baldwin & Co
The oldest herbalist suppliers in London, carrying a
wide variety of dried herbs and pages of advice.
www.baldwins.co.uk

Naturally Thinking
Organic carrier oils, natural beeswax, butters and essential oils, and
also a variety of eco-friendly packaging options for creams and balms.
www.naturallythinking.com

Wares of Knutsford
A wonderful range of decorative bottles, jars and kitchen equipment.
www.waresofknutsford.co.uk

Herbal Haven
Grow over 150 varieties of medicinal, culinary and aromatic herbs (UK only).
www.herbalhaven.com

The Soap Kitchen
Silicon moulds, and lotion- and soap-making supplies.
www.thesoapkitchen.co.uk

Lordington Lavender
West Sussex lavender growers and producers of
pesticide-free lavender essential oil.
www.lordingtonlavender.co.uk

IMAGE CREDITS

NOTES

THE
HEDGEROW
APOTHECARY

RECIPES, REMEDIES
AND RITUALS

CHRISTINE IVERSON

THE HEDGEROW APOTHECARY

Christine Iverson

Hardback
ISBN: 978-1-78783-029-5

*Learn to forage in the hedgerows
like the herbalists of the past*

Discover how to make delicious preserves, healing balms, soothing toddies and cures with nature's jewels such as rosehips, elderberries and mugwort. This sustainable and ethical art is also laced with fascinating folklore and steeped in history. With photographs to help you safely identify edible plants, advice on what is available each season and how best to prepare and preserve your finds, this is the essential guide to enjoying the bountiful delights of the hedgerow.

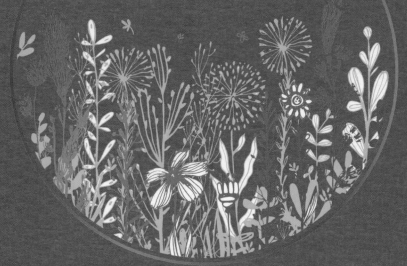

THE
GARDEN
APOTHECARY

RECIPES, REMEDIES AND RITUALS

CHRISTINE IVERSON

author of the bestselling *The Hedgerow Apothecary*

THE GARDEN APOTHECARY

Christine Iverson

Hardback
ISBN: 978-1-78783-979-3

Learn how to make the most of your common garden plants like the herbalists of the past

Unlock the sustainable and ethical art of the apothecarist, and explore its rich folklore and history. Discover the hidden delights in your own garden and how to use them to make delicious edible treats, herbal cures and restorative beauty products. With photographs to help you safely identify edible plants and tips on how best to prepare and preserve your finds, this is the essential guide to enjoying the home-grown riches of your garden.

Have you enjoyed this book?

If so, why not write a review on your favourite website?
If you're interested in finding out more about our books,
find us on Facebook at Summersdale Publishers,
on Twitter at @Summersdale and on Instagram and
TikTok at @summersdalebooks and get in touch.
We'd love to hear from you!

www.summersdale.com